For Fanny Gutiérrez-Meyers

Contents

Acknowledgments

I ARRIVED AT A DIFFERENT PLACE THAN I INTENDED, THEN SOMEHOW found my way back along different paths. There were many people who whispered hints of direction along the way. These good people are Kalman Applbaum, Julien Bonhomme, Jean-François Braunstein, Ed Burns, Jeremy Greene, Erin Koch, Guillaume Le Blanc, Céline Lefève, Annette Leibing, Anne Lovell, Beckie Marsland, Maria Muhle, and Paul Rabinow. Conversations with Robert Desjarlais continually nourish my thoughts and I cannot thank him enough for his intellectual generosity over the past few years. During my time as a student at the Johns Hopkins University I benefited greatly from the encouragement of Abigail Baim-Lance, Thomas Cousins, Jennifer Culbert, Hent de Vries, Clara Han, Ruth Leys, Neena Mahadev, Sidharthan Maunaguru, Sameena Mulla, Ross Parsons, Sylvain Perdigon, Lindsey Reynolds, and Isaias Rojas-Perez. I owe a tremendous debt of gratitude to Veena Das, who helped to shape the ideas in my work in their formative moments.

My colleagues at Wayne State University have been welcoming and energizing, and I would like to particularly thank Sherri Briller, Mark Luborsky, and Andrea Sankar for their support. Fanny Gutiérrez-Meyers inspires daily. There are no greater collaborators, conspirators, and interlocutors than Richard Baxstrom and Stefanos Geroulanos. At the clinic, Philip Clemmey and Geetha Subramaniam opened many doors, even ones I was too tentative to pass through. During the early stages of writing, Peter Quinn and Gillian Stewart Quinn shared their home with me, allowing my mind to breathe a little.

I have benefited greatly from time spent writing and working in France. I was able to present an early version of one of the chapters at the Centre Georges Canguilhem in Paris with an invitation from Pascal Nouvel and Dominique Lecourt. François Delaporte and Sandra Laugier created numerous opportunities for me to develop my thoughts during stays at the Université de Picardie Jules Verne in Amiens. Isabelle Baszanger arranged time for writing at the Centre de Recherche Médecine, Sciences, Santé et Société (CERMES) in Villejuif. At CERMES, I thank Maurice Cassier, Jean-Paul Gaudillière, Ilana Löwy, and Christiane Sinding for their generosity and hospitality. There is nothing quite like the disorientation of another language to make one care for words.

In 2009, Eugene Raikhel, Will Garriott, and Sandra Hyde organized a workshop at McGill University, "Anthropologies of Addiction," where I benefited from the insights of Nancy Campbell, Summerson Carr, Angela Garcia, Helena Hansen, Barbara Koenig, Daniel Lende, Stephanie Lloyd, Dawn Moore, Michael Oldani, and Tobias Rees. Several of the chapters were presented in various stages of development as seminars and lectures in the Department of Social Anthropology at the University of Edinburgh, the École des Hautes Études en Sciences Sociales (EHESS), the University of Michigan Substance Abuse Research Center, the University of Wisconsin–Milwaukee, the Collège International de Philosophie, the Université Bordeaux-3, and in the MéOS (Le Médicament comme Objet Social) research group at the Université de Montréal. I am grateful to the participants at each of these venues for their input. I am also indebted to Jacqueline Ettinger, Tim Zimmerman, Phillip Thurtle, and Rob Mitchell for their keen editorial insights and support throughout.

I have been rich in mentors. Jonathan Ellen has been a driving force behind my work for well over ten years. Throughout the time I have known her, Pamela Reynolds has guided my scholarship gently and sensibly. Paola Marrati's intellectual curiosity has been—and remains—contagious. My conversations with Lori Leonard continually restore my enthusiasm for working and thinking. And finally, the kindness of thought Harry Marks showed to me over the years I was fortunate to know him is humbling. My appreciation extends well beyond what is possible to say here.

In order to conduct my research, I received financial support in many forms. A large portion of the research was supported through a Ruth L. Kirschstein fellowship from the National Institutes of Health (2006–2009). At the Johns Hopkins University, I was awarded a Dean's Teaching Fellowship (2007), the J. Brian Key Summer Research Fellowship (2005), and a Summer Research Grant from the Program for Women, Gender and Sexuality

(2002). I also received ongoing support during the period of research from the Department of Anthropology and the Office of the Dean in the Zanvyl Krieger School of Arts & Sciences. I was able to spend a year at the Bloomberg School of Public Health in the Department of Population and Family Health Sciences with financial support from the Andrew W. Mellon Foundation Population Program (2003–2004). And lastly, I received a dissertation award from the National Science Foundation, Science and Society program (2006–2007), which allowed me to conduct archival research. Without this financial support, I doubt that the following study would have been possible.

It nearly goes without saying that for their openness and trust I owe much to the individuals and families described in the pages that follow. After all the thanks, it is more than a convention that I remind the reader that responsibility for the material presented falls squarely on its author.

A version of chapter 4 appears as "A Few Ways to Become Unreasonable: Pharmacotherapy Inside and Outside the Clinic" in *Addiction Trajectories*, edited by Eugene Raikhel and William Garriott (Durham, NC: Duke University Press, 2013). A section of chapter 5 appears in French as "Le patient comme catégorie de pensée" in the *Archives de philosophie* 73, no. 4 (2010): 687–701. And a small section of chapter 6 appears as "Kevin Is Nowhere" in *anthropologies*, edited by Richard Baxstrom and Todd Meyers (Baltimore, MD: Creative Capitalism, 2008).

THE CLINIC AND ELSEWHERE

INTRODUCTION

The popular medical formulation of morality that goes back to Ariston of Chios, "virtue is the health of the soul," would have to be changed to become useful, at least to read: "*your* virtue is the health of *your* soul." For there is no health as such, and all attempts to define a thing that way have been wretched failures. Even the determination of what is healthy for your *body* depends on your goal, your energies, your impulses, your errors, and above all on the ideals and phantasms of your soul. Thus there are innumerable healths of the body; and the more we allow the unique and incomparable to raise its head again, and the more we abjure the dogma of the "equality of men," the more must the concept of *normal* health, along with a normal diet and the normal course of an illness, be abandoned by medical men. Only then would the time have come to reflect on the health and illness of the *soul*, and to find the peculiar virtue of each man in the health of his soul. In one person, of course, this health could look like its opposite in another person.

—Friedrich Nietzsche, *The Gay Science* (1882)

We step into the reception area of the treatment center, completely bathed in sunlight pouring from the windows. Every smudge on the door and windowpanes glows yellow. The linoleum floor looks as if it's illuminated from within.

Cedric rests against the receptionist's desk, propping himself up on three fingers, his other hand clutching a satchel and several plastic bags filled with shoes, what looks like classroom handouts, and toiletries. "Makes you sleepy," he says. We wait together in the foyer as the social worker and Cedric's mother talk about meeting schedules, exchange documents, and sign last-minute paperwork in hushed but serious tones. Cedric is right; the warm light does make you sleepy. It is too comfortable to pay much attention to the final administrative details being negotiated only a few feet away. Cedric and I stand next to one another, silently, each with our eyes half closed . . .

A white van pulls up along the sidewalk at the bottom of the stairs several feet below the front entrance. A group of young men and women returning from a day-trip marches past us, together with a rush of cool air and the smell of decaying leaves. "Will it be nice not having to do this kind of thing anymore?" I ask, referring to the group that is now heading up the stairwell to a therapy session. "I don't know," he says, "I still gotta take my pills and shit." Cedric, now looking defeated, tells me, "It ain't like I'm really leaving."

THE CLINIC AND ELSEWHERE

Between July 2005 and May 2008, I conducted an ethnographic study of opiate-dependent adolescents in a drug rehabilitation treatment center in Baltimore, Maryland.[1] There, I followed a small group of young men and women from the time they entered residential drug treatment. Once they were discharged, I continued to follow them into their neighborhoods, homes, and other clinical and nonclinical institutional settings—including, too often, back into drug rehabilitation.

The backgrounds of the adolescents I followed varied widely, not only in terms of their economic situations or demographic characteristics, but also in the ways they came to use and abuse opiates, and the paths that eventually led them into treatment. Despite the variation there was an area of experience shared among them, a common element among the therapies they received. They each had either been enrolled in a clinical trial or were currently being treated with a relatively new drug for opiate withdrawal and replacement therapy: buprenorphine.[2] What emerged in my work was a focus on this pharmacotherapy, and specifically two pharmaceuticals developed under the names Suboxone (a combination drug consisting of buprenorphine and naloxone) and Subutex (buprenorphine). Working in a similar way to methadone, Suboxone and Subutex are pharmaceuticals that mirror the neurochemical effects of drugs like heroin, but have the benefit of being more easily and safely regulated in therapeutic doses—with the idea (hope) that, over time, one can be freed from dependence upon other opiates. By engaging in a long-term ethnographic study of treatment, inside and outside the clinic, I sought to trace out patterns of pharmaceutically mediated experience and to better understand the mutual shaping of addiction and treatment for adolescents.

Over the past few decades, the sharp divide between the licit and illicit use of pharmaceuticals has become increasingly blurred, both epidemiologically and through forms of individual reasoning associated with use.[3] Self-medication, the abuse of prescription opioids, and prescription sharing, are all characteristics of use that require a detailed accounting. In the following pages this accounting shows how adolescents do not remain forever institutionally (legally and clinically) visible, one that moves sharply away from a perspective that assumes adolescents' experiences of drug use and abuse to be largely unvaried.[4] Likewise, no single "picture" can provide a satisfactory understanding of the experience of a therapy. Not all of the adolescents I followed lived in unstable households, though many did. Some lived in the suburbs and some in the city. Not all had parents or guardians who were abusing drugs, though there were some. There were some who, in the time I knew them, experienced periods of recovery from dependency, though these cases were few. In the group of adolescents that I followed, patterns of serious drug abuse were episodic and more often described than observed. The ethnography is one in which I contend with shadows and disappearances—*bodies* were not always present or made available (in the strictest sense, as *being present* or *in the flesh*). In the end, there were many distinct bodies: the *therapeutic body*, the *experimental body*, the *absent body*, the *dangerous body*, the *habituated body*, the *medically altered body*, the *reluctant body*, the *recovered body*—and in two cases, the *deceased body*.[5]

I followed twelve adolescents for nearly three years.[6] *Follow*, however, may be too strong a word. At any given time I had consistent contact with three or four adolescents. *Follow* would have to include conversations with concerned family members, friends, parole officers, clinicians, and social workers—often in the absence of the "study participant." Rumor, too, was a form of *following*.[7] Rumors passed between adolescents at the treatment center, between staff members and nurses, and, at home, between friends and family. *Follow* would include documenting the work of clinicians and the material administrative traces that remained after someone would disappear—a *file self*, to use Roma Chatterji's terminology.[8] *Follow* would also need to account for and blend the moments of impaired and unimpaired interaction with adolescents using drugs. As such, the method of retention in the study consisted of multiple phone calls, dropping in unexpectedly, missteps, chance, and very often disappointment. In my work the terms *attrition* and *loss to follow-up*, which are so often heard in human subjects research, do not easily find a place in the grammar of lived experience.

EFFICACY AND EFFECTIVENESS

When an existing pain medication—Buprenex (buprenorphine)—was made available for the treatment of opiate dependence, it marked a dramatic change in public policy directed at the regulation of drug dependency treatment and opened new clinical possibilities for the treatment of a set of difficult disorders relating to drug abuse.[9] Once the drug was approved and the criteria for efficacy in early clinical trials claimed less attention, the long-term clinical effectiveness of the treatment generated concern. The questions asked during a clinical trial are highly circumscribed and are not generally designed to anticipate concerns beyond their frame. To put this another way, the duration of research and the measure of a therapy's efficacy are finite and specific in the context of a randomized controlled trial.[10] And yet there remains a fundamental tension between the efficacy of a therapy during a clinical trial and the clinical effectiveness a drug may have outside the parameters of research, especially within diverse populations outside closely monitored settings.[11]

At its core, the approach of a clinical trial is direct: does some *thing* (either a pharmaceutical or behavioral intervention) satisfy the questions asked of it during a specified timeframe? Of course not every research question can be answered by a clinical trial, or even many trials, just as no one drug is the key to unlocking addiction. The nature of drug addiction is cyclical and lifelong—a disorder or set of disorders as much chemical as behavioral, which carry a tremendous moral and social weight even in the aftermath of abuse.[12] In the case of buprenorphine, the desired clinical outcome of the pharmacotherapy is straightforward: to lessen discomfort associated with withdrawal symptoms, to lessen craving for other opiates, and to eventually reduce the replacement dosage over time. However, patients and their families have other expectations (demands) of the therapy. The evidence of success is not always the same between research and clinical practice, and between the various actors inside and outside the clinic the differences are even more pronounced.

In the case of two adolescents I followed—Cedric and Megan—their fidelity to the treatment regime could withstand (at least in their minds) the use of other illicit drugs in the name of "recovery" or "working to get clean." For the physicians I worked with, having adolescents return to the clinic each week for outpatient therapy, no matter the state they were in, was often equated with a certain degree of success. Just being there, in the flesh, was a measure of therapeutic progress. In each of the cases I followed—between home and the clinic—different criteria for evidence were used to judge the success of a therapy through forms of clinical reasoning that, at times, ran alongside—and at other times completely counter to—individuals' experiences with therapy.

Having said all this, it needs to be made clear that the objective of the book is neither to call into question the criteria for evidence in a clinical trial, nor to claim that the conclusions drawn from the existing research on the efficacy of buprenorphine are false. My aim is to pick up where research questions end—to address other types of questions that emerge through the experiences of individuals under therapy, particularly at the point where the *clinical* and the *social* become difficult to distinguish.

A HISTORY OF BUPRENORPHINE

The residential treatment center and other institutional environments through which the adolescents passed were not the only sites of the study. The archive was another.[13] There I attempted to construct the history of buprenorphine as a *history of the present*, through the multiple and often-contradictory accounts that exist along the meandering path leading to the drug's approval as a therapy for addiction.[14] In addition, I used a large telephone survey with physicians in Baltimore who were authorized to prescribe buprenorphine in order to more sharply render the portrait produced in the archive.

It was difficult to ignore loudly voiced public debates regarding buprenorphine's limits, benefits, and dangers in the local and national media. I have tried to consider these sources as seriously as the scientific research and writing about buprenorphine, largely because the public debates directly influenced how the science of this new pharmacotherapy was interpreted and understood within the environments in which I worked. I have tried to avoid the temptation of aligning an institutional history of a new pharmaceutical with a story about its unintended social and political consequences. To my mind this type of recounting offers unwarranted coherence to the story of buprenorphine's reception in the clinic. Instead, I have attempted to weave these threads together into the career of a therapy—the career of a pharmacotherapy—and to account for its intersections and its afterlife.

The basic narrative of buprenorphine's reception seems at first blush unproblematic. However, what would otherwise be a familiar story of pharmaceutical development in service to an abiding public health concern demands some careful attention when it comes to its details. Stories about public health problems and the activities that go into remedying those problems tend, for whatever reason, to encourage bold conclusions with a retroactive purpose. Many forward-looking accounts of medical progress are often only backward glances through a lens of assumed value, giving false significance to events while posing as neutral retellings.[15] The claims made in the following pages are not so definitive that they can accommodate strong conclusions. The danger is not so much the substitution of fact with fantasy, but rather that retrospective storytelling limits the conditions of fact. In this book I ask very simple questions: If successful outcomes are the point from which the history of buprenorphine begins, then what criteria for success are used? And by whom, and to what end?

When I attempt to casually describe the story that the book tells, I often find myself retreating into the complicated details of pharmaceutical research and development, or, worse, justifying my close attention to the twists and turns in the lives of adolescents through an anthropological catchall concern, *investigations into illness experience*. I am indeed concerned with the experience of illness, and even more precisely I am concerned with how pharmaceuticals have come to mediate that experience—but the following pages are not only about this. The book is about the difficulty of determining whether a pharmaceutical intervention is a success or failure through often-competing sets of expectations held by different actors. It is also about the surprisingly long reach of clinical reasoning outside the clinical environment and into something we call *the social*. And lastly, it is about the way healing finds coherence in individuals' lives over time. The following pages are about all of these things, woven into a mesh that forms the career of a therapy in the clinic and elsewhere.

So with this in mind, I want to preface my ethnography with a brief reflection on the tension between *cure* and *healing*, because, while quite old, this tension rests at the heart of my investigation into pharmacotherapy for opiate dependence and guides my understanding of the potentials and limitations of therapeutics among research science, clinical practice, and the individual experiences of adolescents receiving pharmaceutical therapy.[16] In a way, the book can be thought of as a long essay on the anthropology of therapeutics and the management of life through pharmaceutical intervention.

AN ANTHROPOLOGY OF THERAPEUTICS

The patient's hope of healing and the limits of medical efficacy are at the core of a short essay written by the preeminent philosopher of medicine Georges Canguilhem for a psychoanalytic review in 1978, entitled "Is a Pedagogy of Healing Possible?"[17] Canguilhem's argument can be summarized plainly: of all the objects of medical thought, healing is the one least considered. The claim may at first seem misleading. If healing is not the primary aim of medicine, if it does not form and therefore occupy the highest order of medical thought and practice—resting at the center of all its objects— then what is? Canguilhem makes an important and necessary distinction: healing is fundamentally subjective and individual, following an etymology that includes protection and security, but also *to defend*.[18] Cure, on the other hand, reflects forms of internal change adhering to external validation. Cure is the success of change *within*, verified statistically or otherwise from *without*. Stated simply, cure is a return whereas healing opens onto something new and previously unfamiliar or unknown. Healing does not restore a previously existing order; it does not return to an old norm.[19] As Canguilhem argues, healing is a process of establishing new norms *in* and *of* the body.[20] I attempt to make this distinction clear through my ethnographic account in the following pages.

The hope of healing and the definitions at work in designating cure expose certain habits of thought pertaining to therapeutics. Even in cases where the patient's expectations are not met (medical practice has failed to cure or to reestablish an earlier order), somehow the absence of cure does not necessarily induce doubt in medicine's potential to do so.[21] In reference to the work of the physician René Leriche, Canguilhem writes: "The invalidity of the sick man's judgment concerning the reality of his own illness is an important theme in a recent theory of disease."[22] If one spends much time in clinics, a common refrain heard is that patients often work *against* a given therapy. Even if the expression is borne of frustration, it shouldn't be mistaken for a kind of crassness or professional impotence. I take these statements seriously, not because they chafe my own sensibilities, but because they tend to bind (and not only discursively) a formal clinical perspective with the realities of care—and expose how the reach of therapeutics is imagined.[23] One of the clinicians with whom I eventually became close would often remind me, "adolescents are *difficult* even when they're not using drugs, so we need to keep it all in perspective." The work of getting patients—adolescents—to follow directions was not an easy task for the clinical staff. The idea of "difficulty" somehow became instrumental within a conception of care in the residential treatment center. Difficulty was a term whose meaning would come to rest somewhere between compliance and misbehavior, allowing a degree of ambiguity to remain when problems would arise because patients did not do what they were told to do. The control of terms was not simply an expression of physician authority, but rather something fundamental to a philosophy and teleology of therapeutics as upheld in the clinic.[24]

As I see it, there are two closely related issues at hand. The first concerns the object of speech. Therapeutics can be understood through the forms of speech taken up in the clinic, and the objects this speech adheres to. With time, what becomes clear is how the language of therapeutic offering in the clinic blends pedestrian and professional discourses. The language used to describe adolescents under treatment retained this kind of duality. They were "okay" or "in bad shape," "feeling better" or "feeling worse," "on the way up" or "on the way down," "good enough to 'go out'" or "sick enough to 'stay in.'" Rarely did the slippery slope of "cure" and "healing" enter the lexicon used in the clinic, but it was always lurking somewhere behind other terms. In fact it is between these two speech genres—professional and pedestrian—that the danger of conflating healing with cure resides. If the patient is somehow both the object of medical work and an object of speech (spoken *to* and *about*), then to ignore the discursive registers that hold "what is done" apart from "what is hoped for" would be wrong in the strictest empirical (ethnographic?) sense. In the most practical way, I found myself tracing these specific points of contact or disconnection (the bracketing of the patient off from therapeutics, and not only rhetorically) in order to see how therapy is imagined versus the way it is actually practiced. My anthropological engagement required identifying *where* these touch-points occurred as much as *how* they acted in concert with a philosophy of therapeutics.[25] Despite already sounding too bold, I say all this not in some prescriptive sense, but as a reminder to myself of what I attempted, and continue to attempt, to do in my work.

The second issue is the distinction between individual, subjective health and collective, public health. As Canguilhem rightly observes, if health is equated with the normal it is still conceptualized as a figurative goal.[26] If health is indeed a concept, or even a domain of concepts, then it is a crudely formed concept.[27] Canguilhem asks: "But is it because therapeutics aims at this state [health] as a good goal to obtain that it is called normal, or is it because the interested party, that is, the sick man, considers it normal that therapeutics aims at it?"[28] The moment of encounter between medicine (its custodians and practitioners) and the sick person seems, at least from the outside, to account for the collective enterprise of medicine and the subjective aspects of illness. But how is such an accounting possible? Whose goals are being articulated in the encounter between medicine and the "interested party"—the one who desires to be "led" back to a state of health?

It is simply insufficient to focus on what is said or what is stated as a goal. To paraphrase Virginia Woolf, in sickness language runs dry.[29] Here, Canguilhem can offer an important insight: "It is impossible for the physician, starting from the accounts of sick men, to understand the experience lived by the sick man, for what men express in ordinary concepts is not directly their experience but their interpretation of an experience for which they have been deprived of adequate concepts."[30] Of course "adequate concepts" are precisely what are at stake in conceptualizations of health, particularly when others provide them. What if, when considering the clinical encounter, we interpret the moment when "language runs dry" in the affirmative rather than the negative? One of the adolescents I followed closely—Jeff—

refused the idea that he could "find the right words" to describe the pain of detoxification. Words would not do. And anyway, what purchase does allowing what is said to assume more value than that which is left unsaid—or cannot be said—have, when that which is held in abeyance remains private and preserved? It is strange how speech by those experiencing illness or suffering is often given a kind of valorized position when attempting to understand the medical encounter or the illness experience, and yet the speech of the patient simultaneously remains a point of suspicion. Perhaps the strongest interrogation of this idea comes from Arthur Kleinman's canonical *The Illness Narratives*, though the critique extends to Erving Goffman as well.[31] But somehow the narrative construction of illness has been overly operationalized as an ethnographic *technique* in the most recent work on illness and suffering.[32] Let me be clear, just as Kleinman is clear:

> Illness complaints are what patients and their families bring to the practitioner. Indeed, locally shared illness idioms create a common ground for patient and practitioner to understand each other in their initial encounter. For the practitioner, too, has been socialized into a particular collective experience of illness. Disease, however, is what the practitioner creates in the recasting of illness in terms of theories of disorder.[33]

The *medical subject* is not just a *subject* because she speaks, but because speech creates a "dialectic between bodily processes and cultural categories, between experience and meaning."[34] But it doesn't require a skillful imagination to picture bodily processes that hold meaning that are nonlinguistic or, for lack of a better term, paralinguistic—running alongside other forms of speech or expression.[35] In the same manner, Clifford Geertz draws inspiration from Stanley Cavell when he writes, "If speaking *for* someone else seems a mysterious process that may be because speaking *to* someone does not seem mysterious enough" (emphasis in original).[36] If there is a point here, it is this: the patient's unspoken experience of illness is not partial or incomplete, but instead may be registered elsewhere and in a form other than narrative—in the body and on its surface, through its gestures and its articulations—just as the significance of the encounter with the clinic may itself be registered elsewhere. Nothing *absents* itself in this deprivation of language, but it may be one way to get out of the bind that a reliance on the illness narrative creates.[37]

And what about cure? Cure, at its most basic, derives its meaning from a statistical norm achieved by counting many bodies—but also from the sense of being able to "restore."[38] The individual patient joins the collective by following the path of those before her; otherwise her behaviors and attitudes are perceived to undermine medicine's *potential to perform cure*. The idea that the patient obstructs cure—to hold the patient responsible for failure—speaks to the ethical (economic?) imperative of the clinic *to resolve disorder and suffering*.[39] In the face of failure, medicine is extraordinary only because it is premised on the certainty of predetermined outcomes. It is in the shadow of Canguilhem's assertion that cure can be undermined by the individual that we find important analytical fissures in medical thought, particularly in the context of evidence-based medicine.[40] To echo the Gestalt-era neuropsychiatrist Kurt Goldstein, the individual experience of illness does not dissolve categories of disorder, but rather reshapes them in a way that fails to conform to the contours of an established order.[41] Along these same lines, the subsequent pages maintain a focus on the individual following the clinical and social life of the patient. I do this fully aware that the focus on an individual (or even a few individuals) leaves so many unanswered questions regarding the significance of findings, generalizability, and meaningfulness in the broadest sense. Does *one* symptomatic body—its physiology and psychology, the registers upon which healing and cure are mutually judged, the status and placement of local moral worlds on the individual, and so on—hold meaning for others? As Gilles Deleuze suggests of the writings of Nietzsche, "Illness is not a motive for a thinking subject, nor is it an object for thought: it constitutes, rather, a secret inter-subjectivity at the heart of a single individual."[42] Illness is deeply individual, expressive, and intimate. The focus on the individual is essential not because it privileges singularity over collectivity, nor because it affords—however strangely—uncertainty, but because such a focus simply has the ability to show that generalizations are sometimes unrecognizable when held up against the individual experience of disorder.[43]

Finally, it is important to understand the significance of the word "pedagogy" in Canguilhem's title ("Is a Pedagogy of Healing Possible?")—pedagogy, in the Greek, παιδαγωγέω (paidagōgeō), from παῖς (país): child and ἄγω (ági): lead; literally, "to lead the child."[44] The assumption is that cure can be, in the strictest sense, instructed. In other words, its properties are known and can be transmitted as formal knowledge or learned behavior. Conversely, *leading one to healing* is precisely the difficulty facing clinicians treating drug dependency. The problem is not an abstraction; it resides in the daily decisions clinicians make in practice, as well as the expectations articulated by patients. The tension between *healing* and *cure* is not about nomenclature or semantics: the tension is found in the lifeworlds of individuals and the moral-social world of the clinic. It is a tension that carries with it certain conceptions of life outside the clinic walls, often with no grasp of how agency is both afforded and constrained by life *elsewhere*. Cure and healing divide claims of efficacy (in research) and effectiveness (in daily clinical practice), as well as direct fresh light toward forms of evidence that go into such claims—evidence, quite literally, as *what is seen, what is spoken or attested to, and what is lived.*[45] I am thinking here of the commitment to a philosophical anthropology that Michel Foucault describes:

> For a long time one has known that the role of philosophy is not to discover what is hidden, but to make visible precisely what is visible, that is to say, to make evident what is so close, so immediate, so intimately linked to us, that because of that we do not perceive it. Whereas the role of science is to reveal what we do not see, the role of philosophy is to let us see what we see.[46]

In the pages that follow, I aim to make what is *seen* and *attested to* in therapeutics ethnographically conspicuous by drawing attention to the details of individuals' lives.

The chapters of the book cover broad domains relating to pharmacotherapy and adolescents under pharmacotherapy, and are arranged to build upon one another conceptually, not chronologically. As I mentioned earlier, I see the book as a long essay on the anthropology of therapeutics and the management of life through pharmaceutical intervention, with each chapter serving to color one small piece of the larger picture.

Chapter 1, "New Uses for Old Things," takes as its point of departure the early clinical trials conducted to evaluate an existing analgesic's effectiveness for treating heroin dependency, which occurred in Baltimore, Maryland, around 1978. At the center of the account is a reflection on the nature of evidence in medicine—what goes into securing evidence and what exposes its limits. The chapter introduces some key questions about buprenorphine's development. Despite being such an appealing alternative to methadone, why did it take decades for buprenorphine to be approved as a therapy for addiction? How did it change the way the treatment of opiate dependency was imagined and performed? And perhaps most importantly, what was the population envisaged to benefit from this new treatment option, and did the treatment reach this group in practice? The extent to which adolescents were invoked in the arguments for the approval of Subutex and Suboxone by the Food and Drug Administration (FDA) and by the Drug Enforcement Administration (DEA) is remarkable—though perhaps less surprising when considered against what appeared to be a looming epidemic of prescription painkiller abuse. In these debates, the figure of the adolescent challenged the categorical stability of *the addict* (the ideal type as an adult with a particular career and pattern of drug abuse), and simultaneously created a more stable position from which to argue for medical and societal need.

Chapter 2, "Monasticism," provides some background for the primary clinical site of the research—a former Catholic monastery in Baltimore now converted into a residential drug treatment clinic. The treatment center, much like its previous incarnation, is a space where adolescents retrain their minds and bodies. The chapter reflects on the space of opiate withdrawal through conversations with Jeff, wherein he describes what is seen and unseen, what is felt and heard, and what it means to dwell with the pain of withdrawal.[47] Through interactions with Ty, Devon, and Heather, I consider the formal and informal organization of time, the desire for (and at times, resentment of) structure, and the difficulty of negotiating relationships within the clinic—with staff, nurses, doctors, and other adolescents. The chapter situates the "patient–subject"—her expressions, affects, feelings, and concealments within therapeutic space—and raises questions about the representation of symptomatic and bodily experience in anthropological writing.

Chapter 3, "Appropriations of Care," explores how danger and risk are produced, assigned, and managed in the contexts of both licit and illicit drug use.[48] The contradictory nature of substituting one opiate for another to treat opiate addiction has been widely discussed and debated; moreover, there is a rich historical literature on the paradoxes of (and fascination with) opiate use in America, its fluctuating legal status, medicinal aspects, connection to pleasure, class dimensions, and so on.[49] Replacement therapy represents one form of substitution, a kind of therapeutic mimesis, but what if pharmaceuticals designed to manage postoperative, chronic, and acute pain are used in unregulated ways with therapeutic intent? Does this idea of substitution also get counted as *pharmacotherapy*? The chapter looks at newly created therapeutic spaces in which addiction treatment occurs, as a result of the transition from specialized drug-treatment facilities (such as methadone clinics) to private, office-based settings. The newly enlarged power of the professional community to prescribe buprenorphine has been regarded as tremendously positive. However, with the transition comes an increasing gap between public and private forms of addiction treatment, possibly creating sharper distinctions between populations based on types of drug abused, degree of dependency, and socioeconomic status. Through conversations with physicians in private practice as well as within specialized drug-treatment facilities—along with one adolescent, Laura, treated in both of these clinical environments—the chapter begins to show how "self care" and the care offered in different and sometimes competing settings creates contradictory expectations of individual agency in relation to treatment.

Chapter 4, "Therapy and Reason," is about the way medical concern is shaped by public attitudes toward drug abuse and treatment. When it comes to opiate dependency treatment, there is tension between the ideas of *the licit* and *the illicit*, since treatment involves using one opiate to wean individuals from dependency on another. Opiates used to treat opiate dependency are viewed as safer, or at least considerably less harmful, than recreational drugs used "just to get high." But in public discourse there is often a failure to recognize the complex calculus at work with individual negotiations of harm, risk, and danger when balancing drug use and therapy. In the end, who is at fault when things go awry? Who is responsible when patients *work against* a given therapy or proceed with treatment in ways that are unanticipated or unwanted? The chapter attempts to address these questions by showing how "adherence" and "noncompliance" are factored into clinical reasoning, and how clinical reasoning is itself diverted.[50] The chapter is organized around an account of three adolescents: Cedric, Wayne, and Megan. Their stories demonstrate how forms of clinical reasoning involved in self-medication interweave a sense of social and intimate security, which in turn remakes therapeutics.

Chapter 5, "Patienthood," offers a theoretical reflection on how the category of "the patient" gets taken up in various ways by the adolescents I followed. Through the work of Georges Canguilhem, Michel Foucault, Friedrich Nietzsche, and others, I argue that the patient is neither solely a subject-position occupied by the person experiencing disorder, nor purely an object of medical intervention. Instead, the patient is a *category of thought*. The clinicians I worked with had very clear notions of what (or who) a patient was and was not. But in a similar way, so did the patients themselves. This contest between shared conceptions of patienthood is at the core of the therapeutic process of addiction treatment. The chapter returns to earlier discussions regarding the criteria for therapeutic success and failure, and asks to what extent these criteria come to respond to the lived realities of treatment and care for different actors.

The final chapter, "Disappearances," attempts to shed light on the disappearances of Keisha and Kevin, and to contend with the deaths of Jeff and Tanya. The chapter reflects on early conversations in the clinic between clinicians, social workers, and adolescents regarding their projections about the future. The chapter dwells on *presence* and its transformative power— a presence that is also the shadow in which anthropological work takes place—and considers the extent to which medicine and social science rely on institutions for access to individuals for study, reflecting on the consequences of such reliance, and asking to what degree anthropological engagements can absorb loss.

How does one go about understanding therapeutics once medical work ends? I address this question by exploring the limits of cure, healing, and the claims made to define and differentiate therapeutic success and failure. My ethnographic gaze is fixed upon the intersection of clinical medicine and social life, at the place where medical and pharmacological subjects are constituted under the sign of therapeutics. By joining the details of the history of a pharmacotherapy with the experiences of individuals under therapy, I depict the uneasy path of return to some *previously existing order* (to borrow phrasing from Canguilhem's essay), and I ask "A return to what kind of order?" In doing so I explore the competing criteria upon which medical intervention is judged—for patients, families, researchers, and physicians. The book is a story of one long-established therapeutic process out of which conclusions are drawn, suggesting the manner in which these conclusions themselves *shape* therapeutics. In the end, it is a story of both success and failure, yet one that shows the intricate patterns of relationships and values formed by a novel therapy.

It seems appropriate to begin the book in the very place where Canguilhem ends his essay—where he reaches back into his title and places the idea of a *pedagogy of healing* under intense scrutiny (*Can one be taught to heal?*): "To learn to heal is to learn the contradiction between today's hope and the defeat that comes in the end—without saying no to today's hope."[51]

1 / NEW USES FOR OLD THINGS

A T THE TIME OF THIS WRITING, IT IS ESTIMATED THAT MORE THAN 500,000 people have been treated with buprenorphine for opiate dependence.[1] In the United States, nearly 16,000 physicians have completed the required training that allows them to prescribe the medication to their patients. Since its approval in 2002, buprenorphine has quickly become the frontline agonist treatment for opiate withdrawal symptoms and replacement therapy for opiate dependency in America. In 2010, the approval of a new delivery system in the form of a Suboxone dissolving film has made buprenorphine an even more appealing treatment option for both patients and physicians alike.[2]

When I began my study, I was primarily interested in the clinical effectiveness of buprenorphine. Does the pharmacotherapy *work* to mitigate the symptoms of withdrawal and dependency for adolescents addicted to opiates, whether it be heroin or opioid narcotic analgesics (prescription painkillers) or both?[3] Specifically, I sought to understand what goes into defining a *working* therapy on the side of young patients, especially after their time in closely monitored clinical environments came to an end. My concern has never been to identify why drug abuse persists, or why periods of abstinence from drug use are often punctuated by crises of other sorts. Instead, I want to grasp how value is derived from a therapeutic tool, in this case a pharmaceutical intervention. Slowly, it was the *afterlife* of a therapy that drew my attention; how a "therapeutic career" is lived alongside and comes to characterize continued illicit drug use, relapse, and bouts of institutional presence and disappearance.

AT THE MARGINS OF KNOWABILITY

In nearly every study since 1992, the long-term outcomes of individuals treated with buprenorphine as a replacement therapy have been described as unknown, representing a major research limitation.[4] In the conclusion of a Cochrane report on the use of buprenorphine to manage opioid dependency, the authors suggest that the limitation is not an artifact of existing research methodologies, but a challenge to the analytical possibilities inherent to addiction research.[5] The nature of drug addiction does not lend itself to straightforward forms of *knowing* (the combination of circumstance, motivations, neurobiology, and other unaccounted factors).[6] Certainly within addiction medicine and the recovery community, the idea of "curing" addiction is far from the established nomenclature used to describe successful outcomes resulting from treatment. But at the same time, there *is* some conceptualization of success at play when it comes to pharmacotherapy. Time is one aspect that narrows the idea of success (Does abstinence from drug use occur between given points in time?), and personal forecasting is yet another aspect (Is what was hoped for as a future—by researchers, physicians, patients, parents, and family members—realized?). The answers to both questions, however, are as elusive as they are illusionary. The limitations, in part technical and in part aspirational, are as much an epistemological problem as a clinical question: What are the *limits of knowing* when it comes to assessing whether a treatment works? Where would these limits begin and end?

Some recent scholarship in medical anthropology addresses these otherwise long-standing debates regarding pharmaceutical intervention. João Biehl's groundbreaking work on antiretroviral therapies in Brazil shows how poverty and marginalization are not simply contexts in which medical interventions are performed, but can give value *to* and deprive value *from* emergent therapies, as well as to the lives managed through medical intervention[7]—a set of assertions that Vinh-Kim Nguyen extends by showing how policy decisions regarding AIDS therapies recast political and social relations in West Africa.[8] Adriana Petryna's cautionary work on medical experimentation details the interdependency and variability of ethics and markets in the production of meaningful scientific knowledge derived from global clinical trials research.[9] Andrew Lakoff's study of psychiatric practice and biotechnology in Argentina demonstrates how ideologies transform clinical reasoning, forms of knowledge, and even the objects of intervention themselves.[10] More recently, Angela Garcia's bold and deeply intimate ethnography of heroin use and abuse in the American southwest examines the unexpected ways that drug use and treatment become registers upon which expressions of relatedness (and "a sense of place") are founded and through which dispossession is articulated.[11] While my focus on pharmacotherapy with adolescents under treatment for drug dependency shares many of the concerns found in recent scholarship, I aim to demonstrate the ways the experience of therapy (however fractured) binds the individual *to* the social and the clinical—and to show that the experience of therapy is not simply held apart from the therapeutic ideal defined by clinical medicine or research science, but instead blends clinical reasoning with the social worlds outside the clinic, reestablishing therapeutics from the inside outward.

A METHOD, OF SORTS

It is worth noting the methodological approach used in my study, and its limitations. I attempted to detail the lives of twelve adolescents during their time inside and outside a drug rehabilitation treatment center. The treatment center, an old converted monastery housing approximately sixty-five adolescents at any given time, was the primary site for recruiting adolescents into the study, through either physician or social worker referral. Strictly speaking, I did not use a cohort approach, namely, taking a single group of adolescents from a shared time zero, moving forward collectively over the three years. The clinical criteria for opiate dependency (heroin and/or prescription opioids), as well as treatment with buprenorphine (either in the clinical trial or simply active treatment), was far too specific in the particular clinic population to make it possible to recruit all twelve adolescents at once. Polysubstance abuse did not always mean opiate dependence, and if opiates were being abused, it did not always mean buprenorphine was used in treatment.[12] Instead, I began with adolescents at different points in time over three years.

Once adolescents were discharged from treatment, I used the networks of relationships in which they were already enmeshed to continue following them. The network of friends, family members, custodians and guardians, social workers, parole officers, and so on, provided a kind of connective tissue between the treatment center and the worlds outside the clinic. But this did not resolve the episodic nature of my interactions. While the unpredictability of my engagement was a feature of individual predicaments and collective circumstances, it deserves note. The residential treatment center seemed at first to provide a solid base from which to organize my research activities, but this base quickly became marred by the same insecurity as the world outside its walls. And the world outside the clinic was, to paraphrase Maurice Merleau-Ponty's formulation regarding bodily interiority, *not elsewhere*, but rather the clinic was carried into other places—a kind of intra-corporality between body and place—even if these other places were, in a sense, nowhere.[13] In reflecting on how (and why) this *elsewhere*—this *nowhere*—could merit any attention at all, I am struck by Michael Taussig's recent writings on anthropological fieldwork. He writes,

> They say science has two phases: the imaginative logic of discovery, followed by the harsh discipline of proof. Yet proof is elusive when it comes to human affairs; a social nexus is not a laboratory, laws of cause and effect are trivial when it comes to the soul, and the meaning of events and actions is to be found elsewhere, as in the mix of emotion and reasoning that took the anthropologist on her or his travels in the first place.[14]

This imprecise mix of emotion and reason drove my ethnographic pursuit of adolescents who would otherwise elude regard outside the clinic.

In order to gain access to adolescents under treatment, I became involved in a phase-III clinical trial for buprenorphine-naloxone (Suboxone) being conducted at the treatment center in Baltimore, a trial conducted through the National Institutes of Health / National Institute on Drug Abuse Clinical Trials Network. The trial compared two different treatment approaches to assess the efficacy of Suboxone in a large cohort of opiate-dependent adolescents. The residential treatment center in Baltimore was one of six sites nationally. When I began enrolling adolescents in my study at the Baltimore site, the clinical trial was well underway.

The clinical trial compared two treatment modalities. The researchers randomized adolescents into two treatment groups: a 14-day, direct-therapy group with no long-term psychosocial therapy, and a 12-week group with highly monitored treatment and psychosocial therapy.[15] In the end, while the adolescents in the 12-week group showed better progress initially (fewer reported cravings and a decrease in other opiate use), the most striking result of the study was that there was no difference between the treatment groups at the close of the 12-month follow-up period. There was also better retention in the group receiving more intensive and highly monitored treatment, but once that ended, the groups were indistinguishable no matter the earlier level of intervention. In addition, the researchers reported difficulty estimating the number of patients who achieved recovery, defined as a "voluntarily maintained lifestyle characterized by sobriety, personal health, and citizenship."[16] The conclusions the researchers drew from the study were clear: retention in long-term treatment is a strong measure of the therapy's success or failure, but there is little known about what happens once adolescents leave monitored treatment environments.

During the weeks after the release of the study results, I talked at length with the researchers involved. I had grown to admire several of the clinicians involved in the study—clinicians who strongly supported and encouraged my efforts to follow adolescents beyond the walls of the treatment center and beyond the follow-up period of their study. In a meeting that took place in Baltimore a few weeks after the data were complied, several of the researchers shared their thoughts on the results with me:

[PHYSICIAN]: It's really hard to know what's working and not working. These data say the therapy works, but with a pretty big caveat: time.

[RESEARCH ASSISTANT]: But does it matter? I mean, while the kids were here they did great. When they leave, I mean, what are you going to do? I mean it's really the things we can't control, like mom and dad and friends, or society, right?

TODD: Are you saying these things you mention can't be factored into the reporting?

[PHYSICIAN]: No, that's not what she's saying. It's that it is virtually impossible to capture. You can say, "this kid went to group," or "this kid kept his appointments," or "this kid dropped out," but the details that go into each of these . . . umm . . . mitigating factors are a different question entirely. It's not going to change how I treat kids when they come in addicted, or even leave addicted.

[NURSE PRACTITIONER]: I know what you're getting at, but the study design is just not able to incorporate your ideal situation of being a fly on the wall in the kids' lives, or tracking a thousand little variables that may or may not have anything to do with the pharmaceutical itself. We try to pay attention to that stuff when the kids come in for treatment, but as clinicians, not researchers.

TODD: I'm only saying that it seems like a lot of unaccounted things surely must influence whether or not a kid stays clean in the long haul, and it must be that sometime things break down . . .

[PHYSICIAN]: [Laughing] We're not picking on you, it's just that you need to know what a randomized controlled trial is all about. The drug works—but in the long term things begin to fall apart. That doesn't change standard of care. Of course you're right about trying to capture other factors, but that's a social science problem. Come on, it's your department.

The results of the trial do open up a large "social science" problem, namely, the problem of factors external to a pharmacotherapy that determine its success. There seems to be a serious difference between the *clinical* and *research* lens, but in the end, "it doesn't change the standard of care." When the nurse practitioner who was associated with the study talked about paying attention to the things that surround the receipt of therapy, nondiscursive indications of the therapy's effectiveness (affect, comportment, mannerism) become discursive *things* that are discussed at length every day in the clinic. The fact that the details of a patient's lifeworld cannot find a register in the research is telling. But even more revealing is the way that these are somehow held apart from the research, making them "clinical" concerns in the most abstract sense.

Holding in suspension "the clinical" for the aims of "research" did not present a problem. It is clear that the results of the study, while frustrating, did not undermine the commitment to the pharmacotherapy or challenge the integrity of the clinical trial itself. The researchers staunchly defended the borders that delineate research and treatment. To quote one clinician,

"Research is research, treatment is treatment, and anything outside is outside—it's all about the kinds of questions you ask." The results (and the reactions to the results) brought a key issue to light, namely, that the pharmacotherapy had a secure place within the logics of research and treatment, although long-term experiences by individuals with the therapy were much less secure.

In the end, I had several questions that could not be resolved by the idea that research, treatment, and the experience of therapy could remain neatly parsimonious. What happens to those adolescents who do not complete treatment? Or disappear once the time of research has expired? How should we regard them? And how do these results factor into the evolving narrative of buprenorphine?

NEW USES FOR OLD THINGS

On October 9, 2002, U.S. Senator Carl Levin issued a press release announcing the approval of buprenorphine for the treatment of opiate dependence.[17] The document cited decades of research and a constellation of clinical trials demonstrating buprenorphine's efficacy as a pharmacotherapy for opiate withdrawal and replacement therapy, which had been entered into evidence during congressional hearings on the drug's approval.[18] In the wake of this research, a new addiction treatment was made available—a treatment that renewed hope for thousands addicted to heroin and prescription opioids.[19] The first of these clinical trials had begun over twenty-four years earlier.

In 1978, Donald Jasinski published a landmark paper from a small clinical trial using Buprenex, an analgesic licensed for the treatment of moderate to severe postoperative pain, in an attempt to treat opiate dependence in adults addicted to heroin.[20] Jasinski and his colleagues conducted their work at the Bayview Hospital in Baltimore, one of the Johns Hopkins University medical centers. The participants in the study were by all accounts serious substance abusers. The inclusion criteria included having been addicted for at least four months and the use of heroin two or more times a day. The researchers had designed a randomized, double-masked, parallel group clinical trial in which, over a four-month period, sublingually administered buprenorphine was compared to two different dosages of orally administered methadone, followed by a period of gradual dose reduction and eventually placebo. The two outcome measures of the study were retention in treatment and the presence of opioids in urine samples. At the time, the study was the largest randomized controlled trial demonstrating the efficacy of buprenorphine compared to the standard addiction treatment, which was then methadone. In the end, the researchers found that there was little difference between the groups during the detoxification phase, but that there was greater retention in the buprenorphine group, suggesting that the drug held significant potential as an alternative therapy to methadone.[21] Buprenorphine was not a miracle drug, however it was equally efficacious compared to existing therapies in treating dependency, and its advantage was that it was safer and had a reportedly lower "abuse potential" than methadone.

Over the following decade, a series of randomized controlled trials followed, comparing the efficacy of buprenorphine (a partial μ-receptor agonist) against methadone (a full μ-receptor agonist),[22] as well as trials comparing buprenorphine to placebo.[23] The success of buprenorphine in the context of research suggested that the drug would be a good alternative to methadone, and quickly replaced the attention given to other novel therapies for opiate dependence[24]—and there were certainly other drugs found to have some potential for success.[25] The research with buprenorphine, however, overshadowed these other potential alternative therapies.[26] Nevertheless, *how* to best administer the new therapy (intravenously, orally, sublingually) and at what speed (rapid induction, slow release) remained unclear.[27]

In 1995, a series of studies were collected in a published volume anticipating the approval of buprenorphine for the treatment of opiate dependency.[28] In the same year as the volume was published, Rolley E. Johnson and colleagues conducted another trial at the Bayview Hospital in Baltimore. This was a placebo-controlled trial of buprenorphine treatment, intended to provide further evidence of its efficacy. Despite their efforts, the results of Johnson's study failed to result in FDA approval of the treatment. The treatment was novel and successful, but the novelty of the social concern (and political mobilization) regarding a changing profile of the substance-using populations had yet to take place.[29] Other treatment options besides methadone were in existence, and while these would be prescribed in the same way as methadone, there was little motivation to systematically change the frontline opiate agonist therapy with buprenorphine.[30] Even in the face of public scrutiny, methadone maintenance was the holdout.[31] When Mark McClellan, the commissioner of the FDA, wrote a small article in the *Journal of the American Medical Association* announcing the approval of buprenorphine in 2002, he touched upon the existing problems of heroin abuse, though his emphasis was on the new area of prescription narcotic opioid abuse and the social costs of *this* particular form of abuse.[32] Only after the change in social and epidemiologic focus from heroin to prescription opiate abuse did the FDA chose to approve buprenorphine for dependency treatment, and more specifically the two drugs that Reckitt Benckiser Pharmaceuticals (formerly Reckitt Coleman) developed and lobbied strongly to have approved.[33]

In 2000, the Drug Addiction Treatment Act (DATA)[34] officially rescheduled buprenorphine with the Drug Enforcement Administration (DEA), which allowed physicians to prescribe it privately (albeit in regulated fashion) rather than in monitored treatment settings such as methadone clinics.[35] In 2002, the FDA approved two new drugs developed by Reckitt Benckiser for use in opiate-dependency treatment, Subutex (buprenorphine) and Suboxone (buprenorphine-naloxone). In addition to their approval, the drugs received orphan drug status, a designation given by the Office of Orphan Products Development (OOPD) dedicated to promoting the development of products that demonstrate promise for the treatment of rare diseases or conditions, as well as drugs that address difficult disorders that are nevertheless prohibitively expensive, unprofitable to develop, or somewhat unpleasant for a company to be associated with. In this case, the designation gave the pharmaceutical company Reckitt Benckiser tax incentives and exclusive rights to develop their product without market competition.[36]

BEYOND THE IDEAL TYPE

The efforts that went into testing and approving buprenorphine as an alternative to existing forms of opiate-dependency treatment were tremendous. And yet the success was, in part, due to an increase of adolescent opioid abuse in the United States.[37] In response to the trend, clinicians and researchers attempted to achieve finer-grained understandings of what worked and didn't work in terms of short-term and long-term treatment—and for good reason. In an editorial published in the *Journal of the American Medical Association,* the authors cited alarming national figures: nearly 232,000 adolescents reported misuse of at least one prescription opioid in 2007. In that same year, approximately 24,000 adolescents had used heroin.[38] The proportion of high school seniors reporting past-year heroin use increased from 0.6 percent in 1992 to 0.9 percent in 2007. The abuse of prescription opioids increased from 3.3 percent in 1992 to 9.5 percent in 2004.[39] By all accounts, the impact of prescription opioids (painkillers) on patterns of dependency in comparison to heroin was by no means negligible. The difference in incidences of misuse between so-called *licit* forms of opiates such as prescription painkillers and *illicit* opiates such as heroin may have something to do with easy availability, although in cities like Baltimore heroin is notoriously easy to procure. The categorical distinction between *legal* and *illegal* drugs somehow holds sway despite similar patterns of nontherapeutic use. During my lengthy interviews with parents of opiate-dependent adolescents, a sentiment conveyed repeatedly was that heroin just "seemed worse" than the abuse of prescription drugs. The association between the intravenous use of heroin and the transmission of the human immunodeficiency virus (HIV) and hepatitis C (HCV) did not escape the attention of these parents. While the routes by which adolescents *take* drugs says something about the sharp distinction drawn between heroin and prescription opiates, the adolescents in the group that I followed overwhelmingly denied injecting during the time I spoke with them—in fact, most were adamant about their refusal to inject any drug intravenously, associating intravenous use with "old heads," "fiends," and "junkies." These were addicts of another generation, or so the claim went.

As much as the adolescents I followed had clear ideas about what older "junkies" looked like, there is no doubt that there were popular conceptions of the adolescent prescription opiate abuser (suburban, white, female) and a competing picture of the adolescent heroin addict (male, African American, poor, urban).[40] Despite evidence to the contrary, an imaginary formed in debates about the problems of abuse.[41] In part, such renderings are meant to set the problems of abuse for adolescents apart from those of adults. Certainly the consequences of abuse for adolescents are not the same as for adults. The clinicians I worked with were principally concerned with the severity of neurobiological change that accompanies the transition from occasional, episodic opioid use to habituated abuse and dependence for adolescents.[42] Increased, regular exposure to either heroin or prescription painkillers leads to the fixed clinical phenomena that characterize addiction: physical dependence, craving, and loss of control over drug use.[43] They argued that the adolescent brain is particularly susceptible to the effects of drug abuse, including permanent impairment of decision-making and judgment, perpetuating the cycle of subsequent opioid abuse and dependence.[44] Adolescence (12 to 18 years of age) and young adulthood (19 to 24 years of age) present critical windows for intervention and treatment.[45] The implication was that adolescents who use opiates regularly *become* addicts more quickly than adults. *Becoming* is important not only because of the developmental transition made by the adolescent occasional user into the regular user, but *becoming-an-addict* with little hope for recovery is also important since the threat of this transition with substance-abusing adolescents was central to the arguments behind the approval of buprenorphine.[46]

While efforts to address opiate abuse among adolescents were important in the debates surrounding buprenorphine's approval, the examination of treatment efficacy in adolescent populations occurred well after the new medications were FDA approved. By the time of the change in DEA scheduling and the final FDA approval of the two drugs developed by Reckitt Benckiser Pharmaceuticals, there had been only a one randomized controlled trial of addiction-related pharmacotherapy for opioid-addicted adolescents and young adults.[47] However, in the congressional hearings in 2000, the possibility of administering buprenorphine in the treatment of opiate-dependent adolescents in new therapeutic spaces was something held up as both clinically and socially beneficial. What remains puzzling is that at the time the arguments were made to approve buprenorphine for the treatment of withdrawal symptoms and replacement therapy there was little evidence that the treatment would prove effective in this age group.[48] Not only was it unclear how effective the drug would be for adolescents in the short term, no study had fully examined the implications or realities of long-term treatment.[49] Research science would have to catch up to its promise. It was only much later that researchers and policymakers began to express concern about the results of long-term treatment, calling for a better understanding of activities such as psychosocial therapy and outpatient follow-up that come to influence outcomes.[50]

PUTTING A DRUG IN ITS PLACE

When these two new agonist therapies to treat opiate dependence were approved, several things happened. First, the ability to prescribe treatment in office-based settings abruptly increased the use of buprenorphine in the United States, opening new possibilities for effective dependency treatment as well as new spaces where that treatment could be offered.[51] Second, the approval provided the basis for more specialized and tailored treatment of newly identified groups of users. Not only would adults addicted to heroin benefit from these new medications, but a growing number of adults and adolescents either dependent on prescription painkillers postoperatively or misusing these drugs recreationally could also be identified and treated. In the case of office-based treatment, therapy could be offered discreetly, unlike the directly observed therapy at specialized methadone clinics.[52] The division between public and private spaces of treatment would further distinguish one group of users from another.

The social stigma associated with methadone maintenance programs continues to hold true today.[53] In the early moments of methadone maintenance after the Alcoholic and Narcotic Addict Rehabilitation Act of 1968, a similar promise to that of buprenorphine was made—less risk for overdose, less discomfort during withdrawal, and perhaps most importantly, little risk of abuse and diversion of the drug.[54] Despite the revival of the methadone narrative in the context of buprenorphine—one articulating both *promise* of recovery and *threat* of misuse—the similarities end when the spaces in which treatment is offered are considered. Office-based treatment raises unique concerns about patients and physicians alike; specifically, is care being taken on all sides to ensure that these new medications are not being misused? The approval of buprenorphine complicates the picture of *treatment* as well as that of *the addict* precisely because the means by which treatment is offered can take different forms between public and private medical environments, seen and unseen—and this further complicates how social and medical concerns come to be shaped around treatment. *Where* treatment is located is important, especially when negotiating public attitudes and fears, the scope of research science, and the realities of clinical practice.

BALTIMORE, MARYLAND

Baltimore is important to the story of buprenorphine for many reasons. The loss of the steel industry, the railway, and the port are equally backdrops and catalysts for the problems associated with inequalities in healthcare, a disastrous education system, and violence stemming from poverty and exclusion fueled largely by the drug economy. The social and economic problems faced by the city came to bear on the lives of the adolescents I followed in very real ways. They are adolescents from a generation that has *never not* known the HIV epidemic, or the flood of heroin and other drugs drowning their neighborhoods, or the legacy of failed schools, or family members chronically unemployed or underemployed. In the city, even where such things are not experienced directly, they remain inescapable.

Baltimore is bookended to the east and west by two major urban medical centers: the Johns Hopkins Medical Institutions and the University of Maryland School of Medicine. "Baltimore is a research city," one clinician told me while we sat together during grand rounds at the Johns Hopkins Bayview Hospital. "Drug abuse, violence, and exposure to infection . . . [smiling] you can find experts on both sides [referring to both researchers and individuals suffering from these problems]."[55] His blunt assessment felt crude, especially as we drank free Starbucks and ate gourmet sandwiches provided by a pharmaceutical company sponsoring the seminar. Clearly "both sides" are represented in the city. Baltimore has some of the most well-respected and well-funded researchers, as well as some of the highest levels of gun violence, infectious diseases, and drug abuse in the country.[56]

The city is saturated by research occurring in public and academic medical environments. Within the families of the adolescents that I interviewed, there was always at least one person who had some previous experience participating in medical research. I often found myself explaining my research in contrast to other research that people had encountered. One parent asked repeatedly, "What's the catch?" I couldn't seem to satisfy her question no matter how many ways I tried to explain myself. Finally, she became very literal and asked if her son had to enter some kind of learning program, give blood, "piss in a cup," or take some new drug. I responded flatly, "No, nothing but talking." "Oh, okay, so a psychological test," she said. "No, not at all,"

I responded. "So it's not really research then, so that's fine, I mean, it doesn't sound like he has to do anything," she finally agreed. Despite a bruised ego, I wasn't about to make a case for my research *as research* after she gave her consent to let her son participate in my study. Nevertheless I could not shake the feeling she left with me about what research *is* and *is not*, or at the very least the elements she perceived would commonly go along with participation in medical research in Baltimore.

Medical research is in no way foreign to social life in the city. Along with the familiarity of medical research, *the social* and *the clinical* become obscured and interdependent in the characterization of healthcare problems in Baltimore. Elsewhere I have described how both recent and historical moves within preventive medicine and epidemiology that attempt to incorporate social conditions into an otherwise strict biological basis for understanding disease processes (etiology, acquisition, transmission), suggest that the social and the clinical are implicated in the production of one another.[57] Certain behaviors, as they arise from social conditions, are construed in such a way that they appear analogous to a model of disease etiology—and as such, *curing* social ills becomes inseparable from *curing* disease. In other words, understandings of social life seem to conform to understandings of disease. When disorders like drug dependence reside at the point of connection between the social and the clinical, the job of describing the social conditions that contextualize a disorder becomes precarious. Perhaps it is even more precarious in the case of drug abuse and dependency, since *cure* is fundamentally out of bounds. And yet, the social weight that dependency carries is precisely what held the attention of clinicians and legislators, helping to create the possibility of a new treatment through the perception of a new danger.

LITTLE ORANGE PILLS

After talking about buprenorphine for so long, it should not have been a shock to see the small pile of orange pills spread out on a napkin in a fast-food restaurant located a few blocks from the treatment center. I had been working in the residential treatment center for more than a year before I actually saw someone *taking* "bupe" outside the monitored environment. Ty was sixteen years old when I first met him, several months before the conversation we were having now, discussing an outpatient therapy session that had ended an hour before. He noticed my intent look and handed a pill to me for closer examination. "Breath mints," he said, smiling. Ty counted the pills and returned them to a small plastic bag. I passed him the last pill in silence.

The little hexagon-shaped pills have what appears to be a sword imprinted on one side.[58] At an early point during my time at the treatment center, I made a joke with one of the clinicians that maybe the "sword" imprint was a message from the pharmaceutical company warning that the Sword of Damocles hung over all those taking the medication. My joke was unsuccessful, probably for three reasons: first, in this context I tell jokes poorly, already feeling a little scrutinized in my conversations with physicians; second, he did not recognize (or did not care to recognize) the allusion; and third, as I dug deeper into the hole I had made for myself, I tried to explain my meaning, which is rarely the sign of a good joke. The allusion—which isn't a joke at all—referred to something precarious, a sense of foreboding, the inevitability of tragedy, containing a warning against the assumptions of power and overconfidence.[59] "It's just the opposite, don't you think? The drug gives people hope and we know it works," he snapped. His annoyed tone let me know that our conversation was over.

But I maintain that the actual situation of the drug is not too far off. Something that seems so certain, so powerful and unwavering, "tirelessly right," may come with a dagger looming overhead, suspended by a (horse) hair. One of the things shared among the adolescents I met in therapy was the precariousness of their situations. One thing shared between the physicians offering the pharmacotherapy was their attempt to suspend (remedy) this precariousness. Some of the disconnect arose from the therapy itself (Does it work? And if so, how well?), some of it came from the situations in which therapy was offered (What external factors undermine its effectiveness?).

Each of the adolescents I followed took "the little orange pill," but they each *took* it differently. In the case of a young couple, Cedric and Megan, they had intense confidence in the effectiveness of buprenorphine as a replacement therapy. Jeff was inexplicability lucid when describing the process of withdrawal and his experience with the therapy, although he was desperate to return to a time before addiction. He worked to escape these little pills. He wanted more than anything to be free from addiction (and treatment), which may explain why he was so successful with the therapy and stopped using drugs altogether. The intensity of his treatment experience was matched only by the intense interpersonal violence he experienced, a return to drug dealing, and the end that he eventually met. Devon was not successful at all. He suffered the rise and fall of dependency, illness, and a return to heroin. Heather was awash in the complications of the lives of others and barely aware of the therapy, which remained incidental even as she dropped out of (and back into) treatment. Kevin was gone before he could even really begin treatment. Keisha was forced into the role of caregiver, a mother to own her mother and to her siblings, and remained in treatment as a way of establishing a familial role. Tanya remained under therapy to escape sexual abuse and a life that had been emptied of friends and family. When she found companionship and care in a group of older women, she fell ill and eventually suffered a fatal overdose of heroin. And finally, Laura, who despite being granted every opportunity to do so, could never balance the roles of recovery and independence she had created for herself, staying in therapy only to keep one foot in treatment and the other in serious abuse.

The little orange pills were with them throughout.

In the lives of each of the adolescents I followed, pharmacotherapy played an important role. These roles, however, were vastly different, even if, in some cases, the "outcome" looked the same on the surface.

AFTERLIVES

When I say it is in the *afterlife* of treatment where my study begins, what I mean to say is that questions begin at the epistemological threshold of therapeutics, where *knowing* ends. Surely a therapeutic career continues even when it enters the unknown. By starting from the afterlife of a pharmacotherapy, a different history of treatment is constituted. It is a place where success cannot be taken for granted, just as failure may have different criteria imposed upon it as well. Attention to what happens after treatment is both a methodological and an analytical concern. There are criteria that treatment holds to, namely, that patients have to consume the medication (to put it under the tongue until it dissolves) and remain on the course of medication prescribed to them. But it seems that these criteria would also need to incorporate factors that would precipitate relapse or ongoing misuse, even in the periods when the pharmacotherapy ceases to be used or is used differently than prescribed.

The treatment of opioid-addicted adolescents is primarily detoxification and counseling—and while extended pharmaceutically assisted therapy may not be well understood, the *situations* in which therapy is experienced strongly determine outcomes, in whatever form they take.[60] The tension between what is considered efficacious in the context of a randomized controlled trial, and for that matter evidence-based medicine more generally, and the individual realities of clinical treatment, is a problem faced (and largely managed) by clinicians. The problem is how to make coherence out of therapeutic outcomes that seem outwardly incoherent. This concerns the notion and limits of cure, of healing, and what stakes (and claims) are at work in defining success and failure—and, fundamentally, how the question of time relates to evidence.

Buprenorphine offers the promise of recovery from drug dependency. Where and when (and if) recovery occurs is another matter altogether. As the following chapters aim to demonstrate, there is a range of experiences with the medication—even within groups of adolescents that are otherwise similar—in which the predictive power of research is out of step with the lived realities of treatment. The tenor of the debates that surround buprenorphine is equally hard to predict. Public concerns about the abuse and diversion of buprenorphine seem to reach back into anxieties about methadone a few decades earlier.[61] The next chapters will show how public debate can take a firm hold in the reception of any treatment of opiate dependency—and how those under treatment can complicate the terms of concern.

2 / MONASTICISM

Phenomenology demands that images be lived directly, that they be taken as
events in life. When the image is new, the world is new.

—Gaston Bachelard, *The Poetics of Space*

A LONG A HALLWAY WALL OF THE TREATMENT CENTER HANGS A
small picture of Christ leading a group of his followers along a rocky
path. The print is yellowed and its placement on the wall inconspicuous.
Each time I would pass the image I wondered if it had been intentionally left
hanging because in some way it was representative of the treatment process,
or whether it had simply been overlooked. I wondered if this was the scene of
recovery or merely an artifact of the former incarnation of the place.

Through close attention to three young men and one young woman, in
the following chapter I want to offer a picture of what it is to negotiate transactions between body and space in residential drug-dependency treatment.
In doing so, I wish to reflect upon the conditions that come to form an image
of adolescents under treatment. If, as Bachelard suggests, the world is made
anew through the image, then how one goes about rendering such an image
is crucial.

CLINIC AND MONASTERY

The residential drug treatment center is an old converted monastery—
though "converted" may be an overstatement.[1] Religious imagery can still
be found scattered on the walls and represented in statues that cover the
grounds. The monastery was originally built in the Irvington neighborhood
located in southwest Baltimore in 1868, and, after a fire, rebuilt in 1886. The
parish church attached to the old monastery was built in 1932, and remains
operational today.

To say that the setting feels monastic conveys a sense that is only too obvious. The building is enormous. The halls echo loudly and were clearly designed for a quieter clientele. Large windows cover the back wall of the four-story stairwell, affording a view of what used to be herb and vegetable gardens. The front windows afford an expansive vista onto one of the oldest Catholic cemeteries in the city. The section of the cemetery seen from the top floor contains the graves of hundreds of fallen confederate soldiers. The clinical and administrative offices occupy old cells meant originally for prayer and meditation. The building is austere. I was never once unaware of its former incarnation. Even the old bingo hall was host to nightly outpatient therapy.

But "monasticism" in the treatment center is not only a characterization of its physical features. The adolescents who take up residence in this place are charged with following routines, led through everyday rituals of eating, working, sleeping—their bodies and minds being trained through recitation in group therapy and individual counseling, in service of recovery and rebirth.[2] The center is secluded, an island in the city. Here, adolescents are meant to establish new forms of behavior, new patterns of being, new performances of the everyday, new bodily and mental habits. Such things are inescapable if one wants to succeed in treatment.

DISGUISING DETAILS

The treatment center opened in 1989 as part of an established system of behavioral healthcare programs for adults and adolescents in Maryland. The center primarily serves inner-city Baltimore, although referrals from public-sector agencies (juvenile justice and social services) outside the city were also common. At the center, three basic forms of service are provided: short-term residential treatment, day treatment (partial hospitalization), and intensive outpatient care. The adolescents who populate the treatment center have a high severity of substance abuse and most have had unsuccessful periods of treatment in the past. Many of the adolescents have emotional and behavioral symptoms, comorbid psychiatric disorders, and significant functional impairments.[3]

Roughly sixty-five adolescents stay at the center on any given day, and of these, approximately two-thirds are male and one-third female, ranging in

age from 11 to 20. Despite the wide age range in the treatment center population, my focus was on 14 to 18 year olds. I was interested in adolescents who
were poised at several crossroads—who were at a moment marked by clinical, social, and developmental transitions, and for whom significant changes
were occurring in the trajectory of drug use.[4]

Dependence	Abuse
(3 or more in a 12-month period)	(1 or more in a 12-month period) Symptoms must never have met criteria for substance dependence for this class of substance.
Tolerance (marked increase in amount; marked decrease in effect)	Recurrent use resulting in failure to fulfill major role obligation at work, home or school
Characteristic withdrawal symptoms; substance taken to relieve withdrawal	Recurrent use in physically hazardous situations
Substance taken in larger amount and for longer period than intended	Recurrent substance related legal problems
Persistent desire or repeated unsuccessful attempt to quit	Continued use despite persistent or recurrent social oar interpersonal problems caused or exacerbated by substance
Much time/activity to obtain, use, recover	
Important social, occupational, or recreational activities given up or reduced	
Use continues despite knowledge of adverse consequences (e.g., failure to fulfill role obligation, use when physically hazardous)	

In using the DSM-IV criteria, one should specify whether substance dependence is with physiologic dependence (i.e., there is evidence of tolerance or withdrawal) or without physiologic dependence (i.e., no evidence of tolerance or withdrawal). In addition, patients may be variously classified as currently manifesting a pattern of abuse or dependence or as in remission. Those in remission can be divided into four subtypes -- full, early partial, sustained, and sustained partial -- on the basis of whether any of the criteria for abuse or dependence have been met and over what time frame. The remission category can also be used for patients receiving agonist therapy (e.g., methadone maintenance) or for those living in a controlled drug-free environment.

American Psychiatric Association. Diagnostic and Statistical Manual of Mental Disorders. 4th edition (DSM-IV). Washington, DC: American Psychiatric Association, 1994.

Table 1.   Diagnostic and Statistical Manual of Mental Disorders—IV: Criteria for Dependency and Abuse.

The ethnic composition of the treatment center is roughly one-third African American and two-thirds Caucasian. The primary funding source is Medicaid, followed by commercial insurance (Blue Cross/Blue Shield, HMOs), Juvenile Justice (for adolescents in their custody), and other supplemental funding for uninsured or underinsured adolescents. In the population, the majority of adolescents have family and educational problems. On average, only 53 percent report currently living with a parent, and only 29 percent are in school.[5]

In terms of substance use patterns, most adolescents in treatment are high-frequency users and many are daily users. Approximately 96 percent have used substances on 15 or more days in the 90 days preceding admission.[6] The majority of adolescents (91%) meet criteria for the full syndrome of substance dependence (see Table 1). Most of the adolescents (71%) have had one or more prior treatment episodes. Nearly half (46%) have participated previously in residential treatment.[7] In addition to the treatment of substance-use disorders, many of the adolescents require medical monitoring for conditions associated with drug use, as well as preexisting medical conditions unrelated to their drug use. As such, each adolescent is screened and treated for medical complications such as hepatitis, tuberculosis, HIV, and other sexually transmitted diseases.

While the administrative workings of the treatment center are highly ordered, the daily realities faced by administrators and clinicians are unpredictable. Elaborate strategies are used by intake nurses to keep adolescents in treatment. There are long negotiations between parole officers, outside social workers, parents, and guardians to determine the duration of a placement at the center, and what criteria will be used to assess whether an adolescent will stay or will find help somewhere else. The residential staff members do not typically stay employed long, and the turnovers affect the continuity of treatment since the staff have the most sustained contact with adolescents while in treatment.

BUILDING FACTS

Some undeniable facts about the treatment center have to be taken into account in order to understand what happens within its walls. It is loud. It is old. It is cavernous. There are activities seen and unseen. There are spaces that are open, and others completely off limits. The activities that take place (counseling, medical treatment, family visits, sleeping, eating) are each configured in space differently. Not the least of these *facts* are the adolescents as actors within the space. But once these facts are established, it is hard to know what to do with them, how they come to rest upon one another.

Maurice Merleau-Ponty, in his writings on phenomenology and the structure of behavior, suggests a general principle for understanding *facts*: "We will study facts, not in order to verify some hypothesis that transcends them, but to give an internal meaning to the facts themselves. Of utmost important will be the rigor with which one embraces the totality as well as the details of certain facts."[8] The internal meaning of facts at the clinic is difficult to establish. They seem woven together throughout the day, *within* and *between* the space and the actors in the space. The sensory order of the clinic is not something peripheral to an understanding of the place itself; the *sense* of the place figures centrally in how treatment is experienced—its *fact-ness*.

The senses are central to drug dependency, at least in terms of how bodily experience is recounted. Michel Serres describes the senses as the foremost means whereby the body mingles with the world and with itself.[9] The body is not empty, waiting to be filled up with meaning. Along similar lines, Jean-Luc Nancy writes, "The body is already filled up with other bodies."[10] Jeff, whom I first met in the intake office, remained in treatment for several months, "finding his place" in the clinic and its daily routines before returning to the streets. He was someone who described his bodily experience of withdrawal in the greatest detail. Jeff recounted the symptoms he felt in the physical manifestation of withdrawal, confined within the space of the room to which he was led after I had first met him. He had gone through withdrawal more than once in his short life, though he insisted that there is no comparison between the experiences. Jeff eventually found order in the treatment center, which helped him maintain his own felt order. The clinic and its routines provided an anchor and a shield against the threat of a loss of meaning, or, more specifically, the encroachment of thoughts, circumstances, bodily sensations that would cause him to reestablish patterns of drug use and violence (at least for a short time). It is an oversimplification to consider therapeutics as existing only in the activities within the space that defines them as such (the psycho-social counseling, monitoring, or prescribing of medication). Therapy is held by space.

SENSES AND ROUTINE

The first thing I noticed on my initial visit to the treatment center was the sound. I actually noticed it most on my way out, in its absence, as I stepped outside to the parking lot. My ears were ringing. The noise within the old converted monastery echoed sharply through the halls and stairwell, and was felt deep inside my head. The noise at any given time produced a state wherein I was always on the verge of a headache. The sound had a utility, too: it signaled when classes at the day school were changing, when groups had ended, when the residents were going to lunch or dinner, when fights would break out, and when I could intercept people as the day progressed.

The sound was evidence of the many routines at the treatment center. In the corridors, I would find residential staff waiting for the next part of their day to begin. Outside, small groups of staff and caseworkers would smoke and chat while checking their watches, waiting between group meet-ings, classes, and therapy sessions. It was only in these rare, quiet times "in between" that I could ask about the adolescents that I was following. I would receive brief reports, which almost always began with some general assessment of behavior—someone was either "acting okay" or "acting out." The statements were framed as therapeutic assessments, but were largely descriptions of interactions with the staff. Megan, for instance, disliked the staff completely and unapologetically. She would joke with me that she needed to get high just to deal with the "fake doctors" and "wannabe par-ents" that the residential staff came to represent to her. She would pick fights with the staff to "get put away for awhile" so she wouldn't have to "look at they 'old head' faces" ("old heads" referring to the fact that many of them were former addicts). Megan hated the daily routine of the treatment center and would do nearly anything she could to extricate herself from its hold over her. I am convinced that her agreement to talk with me mostly had to do with interrupting the predictability of the day.

I had my own difficulties with the residential staff. My ambiguous status at the treatment center and general comportment as an outsider set me out-side the realm of authority. "Do I have to talk with you?" was the greeting I received when I tried to engage a small gathering of female residential staff in conversation between group sessions on my first day at the treatment center. The matter of other people (including the physicians) not knowing what the "kids are really about" was a refrain I heard during my conversations with staff members. There was a form of insider knowledge to which I (and others) seemingly had no access.

Many of the staff members had experiences with substance abuse in the past, and would talk about these experiences openly with the adolescents under treatment. There seemed to be a privileged relationship between the residential staff and the adolescents at the clinic through a commonality of experience. But the relationship was not without limits. During a fight in the stairwell of the main building, several staff members attempted to separate two girls who had hold of each other's hair. The girls thrashed against the windows on the third floor landing, screaming, slurring obscenities, and kicking wildly. As the girls were being separated, the tiny girl who was one half of the fight said something to the middle-aged African American woman holding her apart from the other girl. It was hard to know what she said over the din of the cheering crowd of onlookers, though the reaction her words provoked was clear. The woman began to lunge toward the girl, and was held back by one of the younger male residential staff members. The middle-aged woman had a look of anger frozen on her face even after the girl had been taken away, presumably to one of the unoccupied rooms on the corridor.

My curiosity about what was said during the exchange between the staff member and the girl stayed with me all day. It was a bit of drama, not too out of the ordinary, but a welcomed break from the routine to which I was subjected as well. I found myself wandering through the halls, loitering in the caseworkers' office, hanging around the front desk, and pacing outside during smoke breaks, hoping all the while that some gossip about the incident would come my way. Eventually I had to ask. "Oh that? That little girl is real close to [name of the residential staff member]. Then [the name of girl] went and said some shit about firing shit up, you know, and it just set shit off," one of the older caseworkers told me between drags of his cigarette. More specifically, the girl said that they should "fire some shit up" referring to intravenously shooting heroin, for which the staff member had been clean and in recovery for over three years. The fight with the other girl had to do with a "new boy" who had been recently admitted, and the "skinny white girl" felt the other girl was trying to thwart her attempts at romance. But romance had nothing to do with what was said to the staff person; it was the intimate knowledge of her own history of substance abuse that was being used to undermine her authority as she broke up the fight.

The fight was not at all remarkable, or even rare, except for this one small detail. The intimacy between staff and the adolescents was used to build trust and to keep the adolescents "under control," though it ran the risk of being used to disrupt the order it was meant to maintain. Devon was one of the adolescents I met who desired the order offered by the treatment center very deeply. The formal and informal organization of time in the treatment center, the way the day and night were scripted, was a necessary part of his stability. He told me:

> I don't want to have to think about being here, doing stuff, talking all damn day about your "drug of choice," messing with people. You just follow along and you can turn off your mind. I like just going with the flow, you know?

I asked Devon about the fight in the stairwell, which I knew he witnessed because I could see him hanging over the railing on the floor above:

> Stupid shit. Just get on with it! Go to class. Go to group. Fuck it. People act like this is real life or something. It ain't. I mean, fuck it. Do what you got to do and get on with it.

Devon was constantly exasperated by things he perceived to disrupt his day, even the otherwise entertaining "cat fight" and the drama of seeing a staff person lose her composure.

The commotion of the fight was nothing compared to the general loudness of the place. How could Devon enter the daze of going through the motions in the course of the day with such acute sensory overload? As I took three aspirin, I presented Devon with a question phrased as a statement: "You can hardly tell anyone is fighting or trying to run away, the place is so loud all the time." Devon raised his eyebrow. "What you mean? Yes you can." He went on to explain that it wasn't the same kind of sound, that you can tell when people are just joking around and when something "real" is happening. The sound that followed Devon was white noise, and its variation wasn't hard to pick out. I asked him if it ever got quiet:

At night, when people finally too tired to mess around, you can feel it.
It's like too quiet, you know. I try to fall asleep before people stop mess-
ing, or I start to think and my mind start hurting, and I want to, you
know, smoke a blunt or some shit. I know it sounds fucked up, but I can't
stand the quiet, like I'm a victim of trauma, like them dudes from Viet
Nam, you know? You *need* that sound of gunfire and choppers and shit.

It is important to pause for a moment on the word "trauma," and for a
specific reason. The word at some point entered the everyday nomenclature
of the treatment center, and became steadily used with such intense frequently by staff and residents alike that the meaning was completely diluted.
"Trauma" and "PTSD" (Post-Traumatic Stress Disorder) were terms offered
to explain (and resolve) everything—in the past and present.[11] This is not to
say that psychological and physical traumas were not very much part of the
experience of the adolescents in treatment. However, not being able to *endure
the quiet* was something that had a different meaning, one that seemed to
resonate with a great many of the adolescents I spoke with at the treatment
center. As much as I would use the sound as a guide to know where the
activities of the day were occurring, as the shouts and laughter reverberated
between the old monastery walls and the walls of my skull, Devon used the
sound as a way to ground himself. The noise *was* the routine, and without it
Devon was left with nothing but the interiority of his thoughts.

ENCOUNTERS

I met Devon, Jeff, and Ty—in one way or another—on the same day. Fit-
tingly, I chose this particular day to sit in the intake room in order to relax,
to drink coffee, and to chat for hours on end with the intake nurses. Spending the day in the intake room felt safe and unobtrusive—restful even.

Devon sat in the reception area for an hour with his mother and a caseworker. He was seventeen years old at the time and had recently returned to
his mother's house, located on the near Westside of Baltimore, after a brief
stay in a juvenile criminal facility in the county. I drove past his house twice
a day nearly every day, coming and going to and from the treatment center.
When he was discharged three weeks later, checking in on him became
part of my daily routine—even if "checking-in" meant glancing over at his

mother's row house to see if there were signs of life. I would stop by every week or so, hoping to catch Devon between the frequent odd jobs (fast food, cleaning, collecting scrap metal, lawn keeping) that he would take on for quick cash.

Devon had been smoking heroin in addition to his regular habit of marijuana for several months. After he and his friends had been caught smoking in his mother's house, she convinced him to go into treatment, though *convincing* took the form of a threat to kick him out of her house if he thought differently. "He was heading down the same road as his father," Devon's mother told me nearly a year after our initial meeting in the lobby of the treatment center. She explained that both Devon's biological father and his stepfather had died in circumstances related to heroin abuse. Devon's father was beaten to death by a group of teenagers when Devon was only three years old. His mother remarried only to be widowed again five years later when her husband died while in a coma brought on by his diabetes. He had been injecting heroin on and off during the five years of the marriage, and Devon's mother associated his death with drug abuse and not diabetes, although it was clear from our conversations that his diabetes was out of control.

Devon sat slumped in his chair, almost horizontal to the floor with his legs spread widely. The female intake nurse asked him a series of questions about allergies, medications, and some demographic information, all while taking his blood pressure. His use of opiates was relatively recent and relatively limited.

After a short stay, Devon was discharged from the treatment center. It had been three months since I had last seen him, during our brief discussions at his mother's house. His mother called to say that he had been admitted to the Sheppard Pratt psychiatric hospital on Baltimore's north side. The day she called was the day of his discharge, and I offered to drive her to the hospital to pick him up if she needed a ride. She accepted and we spoke in the car.

"He so mellow, you know? It's all his weed smoking. And then he just get possessed," Devon's mother told me. She had no idea what triggered the bout of violence that lead to his admission into the psychiatric hospital. He had been picked up by the police, taken to the emergency room for injuries after an assault, and from there was admitted into the psychiatric unit at the Johns Hopkins Hospital. A day later, he was sent to the Sheppard Pratt psychiatric hospital for an unspecified amount of time. Though she had to consent to his hospitalization, Devon's mother was oblivious to the details of his commitment.

I waited in the car as Devon's mother went into the hospital to collect him. After several hours, she returned with Devon, who looked tired and shaken. "Can you just drive us home?" she asked in a tone that told me that a conversation about Devon's psychiatric hospitalization was not welcome.

Devon was silent during the ride back to his house. He stared blankly out the window. Devon's mother also sat in silence. When I deposited them back at their home, Devon simply turned and walked off down the street, leaving his mother watching him from the front steps of the house.

RECORDS

I was told by a caseworker that someone had been admitted over the previous weekend that I might want to talk with. During the early part of the day I attempted to find him—Ty—in the main building. I searched the usual places (day school, nurse's station, counseling rooms) without success. I decided that maybe his chart would give me a clue as to where I could locate him.

It is amazing how quickly an image about a person becomes fixed in one's mind by simply reading their medical chart. The clinical and psychosocial assessments are in no way neutral. They hold a prescriptive power—a clinical picture that is not only clinical. I learned that Ty was a regular alcohol and marijuana user. He had been using prescription opiates on and off for two years. He was arrested and charged with the same offense three times, though the details of these arrests were absent from the file. Ty lived with his aunt. He smoked cigarettes, apparently one pack a day. He had childlike handwriting, based on the many "contracts" he signed regarding his goals for treatment. He was HIV positive. He lived in Baltimore.

Five days passed before I found Ty *in the flesh*. He had been in detoxification, which reportedly had not gone well. When I finally had the chance to sit down with him, Ty was reluctant to talk. He would look at the floor and direct his speech toward his stomach, with his chin resting on his chest. Whenever I asked him if he'd rather not talk to me, he would say it was fine and that he was "okay."

The content of our conversations inside and outside of the clinic was always stunted and remained focused on immediate problems. Inside the treatment center he would be angry and fight with other adolescents. He would complain about the attitude of the nurses. He suspected a younger adolescent resident of repeatedly stealing his cigarettes. Outside the center, he would talk incessantly about being disrespected in various public situations throughout the day. The conversations often felt like a form of misdirection—with things being said so that other things would not be said. Or if details were offered in earnest they were buried beneath layers of passive, detached subterfuge.

It was only after his aunt became ill that he began to bring up his addiction in our conversations, as well as the problems he faced as someone who was HIV positive. He said that he "hated being a drug addict." He also "hated the looks" he'd receive when he'd go in for treatment and medications at the HIV clinic. Seeing himself as an ill person undermined the self-image he wanted to craft. He was desperate to gain "respect," to be seen as a "thug." He wanted to be feared, but by whom and for what reason was unclear. There was evidence that he was largely unsuccessful at this, and most of the time he kept to himself in his aunt's house. He told me, "I don't mess with peoples. I got too much on my mind, and I'd just fuckin' go crazy on people if they bother me." But even statements like these were conveyed unconvincingly. We never discussed many of the things I found in his chart, and only later, when he was threatened by the loss of his aunt, did I realized these were the details that rendered his life profoundly fragile.

HEATHERS

Looking back through the charts from the clinical trial conducted at the treatment center, I found three separate files for Heather. Each of the files had a Polaroid stapled to the inside cover. I laid the three files out to look at the images. Heather seemed to look increasingly better between each photograph. It wasn't until I looked at the dates in the charts that I realized that my assessment was completely backwards. She became progressively thinner—sickly and gaunt—in the images. In the last photograph, that I had mistaken for the first, she was not even looking toward the camera, somehow unaware of its presence, or perhaps just too impaired to care.

I came to know Heather only during her final stay in residential treatment and for a few months after. She then disappeared into the juvenile justice system, and it was impossible to maintain contact with her. Only through the clinical staff did I learn, months after I had lost contact with her, that she had been sent to Delaware to live with relatives. She then returned to Baltimore to stay with a foster family.

Heather desired structure. But more than that she conveyed a desire for connection. The treatment center offered order and a sense of belonging. Treatment was calming, a respite from a world outside the treatment center about which she only hinted. She knew other people were there, always willing to be a part of her life. The treatment center was a place of return no matter in what state she found herself.

Heather said that the times when she was "in between" treatment were when things turned out badly for her, yet to be "outside" was what she most desired. She had been using prescription pills with a much older boyfriend the first time she was admitted for treatment. By all accounts, Heather was consumed with her boyfriend. The arc of the conversations we had began and ended with an account of her relationship with him. "Is treatment working out?" I would ask. "Yeah, my boyfriend thinks I need to get clean for a while. I was getting too hard to handle." She plotted her next move in relation to him. "My mom hates him, but [name] says I can move in with him when I get out." The clinical staff also voiced their deep concern about the force of Heather's romantic entanglements on her treatment.

The Polaroids of Heather are a better record than any clinical assessment could ever hope to provide. By her third admission to the treatment center she had bleached her hair until it was nearly white, and this, with her pale, sunken face, made her appear ghostly. When I tried to talk with her there were times she would lack the capacity to hold a conversation or to engage beyond "yes," "no," or "I don't know." In one of our last conversations at the treatment center, I asked about her boyfriend. She just looked at the floor: "I don't know." Later, one of the nurses mentioned in passing that her boyfriend "got locked up, and when he came home, just left her ass." By the time she was discharged from the treatment center, the image she had constructed for herself through her boyfriend could no longer sustain her. She was adrift.

JEFF

Jeff was one of the adolescents whom I followed closely, and then abruptly lost. When I first met him he was pale, bruised, and sweating. He attempted to sit stoically in a chair in the intake room. I offered him a soda. I watched him hold it without drinking it until he was carried off to detoxification. The nurses shook their heads disapprovingly. "This is not the last time we'll be seeing Mr. [last name]."

It would be.

So much of what went on at the treatment center was about reestablishing order, beyond the rhetoric of achieving "recovery, defined as a voluntarily maintained lifestyle characterized by sobriety, personal health, and citizenship."[12] The core objective was *being well* or *getting well.* But the process was not *reordering* but "ordering"—about creating a new state. Kurt Goldstein writes:

> Being well means to be capable of ordered behavior which may prevail in spite of the impossibility of certain performances which were formerly possible. But the new state of health is not the same as the old one. Recovery is a newly achieved state of ordered functioning, a new individual norm.[13]

The process of withdrawal is one in which someone is "led [pharmacologically or otherwise] . . . through a period of chaos, gently, until he can reestablish a new organization, construct his world anew."[14] The achievement of a new individual norm is not one prescribed from without; it is one that is found *within* the individual. It is unclear in the case of opiate dependence when the "period of chaos" begins. In Jeff's withdrawal, it was the absence of opiates that brought on the sweats, the nausea, and the pain—a certain chaos. When he was using, he described his body as silent ("my shit's quiet").

Silence has its own genealogy in relation to health. Georges Canguilhem returns again and again in his writings to the formulation by the physician René Leriche: "Health is life lived in the silence of the organs."[15] Canguilhem gives intense scrutiny to Leriche's assertion in a forceful essay on the philosophical foundations of health.[16] If health were defined only in the state of its absence, how would we begin to understand when a new norm has been established? In Jeff's case, this silence—the time that he was using heroin and prescription painkillers—was deemed by others to be dangerous and pathological. For Jeff, it was silence that needed to be remedied to make way for health. Michel Serres, writing on the senses, asks, "When a body will not remain silent, what voice do we hear? Comfort, pleasure, pain, sickness, relief, tension, release—noises whispered or wailing?"[17] Serres, following Canguilhem, tells us that silence is at the center of healing, yet this silence tells us nothing:

> Whatever pain or fatigue might ail our body, suffering a thousand ills, overwhelmed by work and injury, it always manages to raise a protective wall around an untarnished space to which the instance of self, quivering with joy and expectation, can flee ever-present danger and imminent death, no matter how far or deep their blows may reach. It starts over, secreting or building a new wall each time an outer barrier is brought down or given up . . . shouting towards silence.[18]

The question remains: *How does one represent the absence of something, even (and especially) to oneself?* If silence forms this veil between illness and health, holding a double meaning or two sets of values between the normal and the pathological, then its representation is important (and remarkably fragile). Representation is important because it is where the contest of value in illness lies. Representation is fragile because the threshold between health and illness in relation to drug dependence is so thin.

REPRESENTATION AND FIGURATION

In 1981, Gilles Deleuze wrote a highly original examination of the work of the English painter Francis Bacon.[19] The book's subtitle, *The Logic of Sensation*, spoke to the conceptual core of Deleuze's analysis. Deleuze was interested in the way Bacon's work moved away from strict representation toward "the Figure" in an attempt to convey "sensation" directly through his paintings.[20] In Bacon's paintings, the human body as a Figure acts as the physical scaffolding that holds in place a precise sensation. Bacon struggled with how to paint sensation—*to record its fact.*

The problems related to sensory experience are simultaneously problems of representation: How is sensation pictured, visually or otherwise? Shigehisa Kuriyama, in his writing on touch in Chinese medicine, describes sensation from a medical standpoint as defining bodies themselves, since sensations were the ways in which living bodies were experienced.[21] Sensation and the form it took in the descriptive language of illness *formed* the medical object. What Kuriyama points out is a move away from generalized notions of bodily experience in relation to disturbance, and toward a view fixed in the corporeal "present tense" of symptomatology. Deleuze identifies similar investments in the paintings of Bacon, where a variety of *experiences of the world* could arise from the same source. In Bacon's paintings, there are relationships between Figures that do not necessarily rely on narrative, which "spring from the same fact, that would belong to one and the same unique fact rather than telling a story or referring to different objects."[22]

Deleuze saw in Bacon's paintings an insistence on presence—on making something visible that is already there in the Figure. Similarly, Michel Foucault's notion of philosophy is precisely about rendering visible what is already there: "to make visible precisely what is visible, that is to say, to make evident what is so close, so immediate, so intimately linked to us, that because of that we do not perceive it."[23]

The conversations with the young men and women I followed were reminders of the impossibility of "telling" certain forms of experience, of the limits of narrative to reproduce (represent) bodily experience. Like Bacon's paintings, which delimit the space where his bodies reside (by creating round areas, drawing them in boxes, locating the Figures in rooms and upon objects like chairs, beds, and rugs), my attempts to capture the process of opiate withdrawal utilize the same methods of delimiting—and "feel" the same constraints, and encounter the same dilemmas.

SPACES OF FEELING

Descriptions of the rooms where detoxification would occur were given to me. I did not enter these spaces; others described them. The rooms are found in a newer section of the treatment center, in a separate, two-story building called the residential hall. The low-ceiling rooms contained cots, chairs, brightly painted walls, a small table, and blankets. The descriptions could easily have been of *any* room. I never ventured into the rooms. Even now, my recounting fails to convey the lasting affective power these descriptions retained for the individuals who spent time there. The place of memory was held onto tightly, and to offer an objective description would seem to betray a trust afforded to me in just being able to hear the descriptions. And why do I care what the rooms were *actually* like anyway? As the symptom of a fetish for the empirical? The sense of the rooms during these particular events was all that mattered. *Witnessing* the space without this sense of space was a great temptation—a temptation to complete the story by offering "the facts" of my own account, to fill in the gaps, to substitute or confirm details, to resolve the contradictions and departures from fact that arose between the stories I was told. In the end, I did not care about facts for their own sake—I cared for what facts did.

Jeff described in great detail the symptoms he felt through the physical manifestation of withdrawal, confined within the space of the room. Jeff had gone through withdrawal more than once, though he insisted that there is no comparison between the experiences. He told me, "It's not like you get good at it. It's like someone who been in a bunch of car accidents, it's not like they say, 'here we go again.'" The physical manifestation of opiate withdrawal is generally not life threatening, but what Jeff's account shows is that it threatens the intactness of life. Life is no longer taken for granted; the process thrusts a person "between living and dying," as he described it to me.

At the treatment center, pharmacological treatments (specifically buprenorphine) are used during acute opiate withdrawal. In addition, a special effort is made at the clinic to provide supportive care and comfort. Some of the adolescents require fairly intensive medical management of their withdrawal symptoms. The nursing staff members explained that there are symptoms they nearly always expect: agitation, tachycardia, hypertension, nausea, vomiting, sweats, diarrhea, irritability, and anxiety. I asked if the list would include pain: "Well, of course!" The onset of withdrawal generally coincides with the time of the next habitual drug dose, which for many occurred well before they entered detoxification. In Jeff's case, withdrawal symptoms set in quickly four hours after the last time he used. He was using less than a gram of heroin daily, as well as some Vicodin, some Oxycontin, drinking alcohol (malt liquor), smoking cigarettes, and consuming "energy drinks" (specifically the energy drink Red Bull). His pulse was racing. I stood at the nurse's station and asked how Jeff was doing. The nurse read off a laundry list of symptoms: "He's restless, he can't stop yawning, he used a whole box of Kleenex blowing his nose, his pupils are dilated, but he's okay." When she felt his skin she told me it was "nothing but goose pimples." Until that point, he had only been given Tylenol on the transport over to the clinic. She tried to reassure Jeff that he'd be "fine by morning." He sat up and tried to drink from a glass of water, but he began to drool and spit it up.

On the second day, he was badly dehydrated and continued to vomit. He stood, and fell immediately from the rush of blood to his head. He stayed in the bed in the fetal position.

Jeff was well-informed about withdrawal and lucid in the description of his experience:

JEFF: The nurses have no idea how scary they get when you're laying there, all soaked in your own sweat, freezing. I'd hear them laugh in the hallway and think, "they're making fun of me." Sometimes I'd think, "they going give me fake drugs to keep me feeling like shit, to teach me a lesson." The biggest gangster'd be like a little kid when you're feeling all that kind of pain. It's not like you shot or something. It's not pain like someone just beat your ass and you're like trying to stay strong. It's like you don't got muscle anymore. You weak.

TODD: Suboxone can make you feel sick in a way that mimics withdrawal. But they change the dosage to make the symptoms less and less, right? [Somehow, offering a quasi-clinical explanation felt safe, if not a little pathetic.]

JEFF: I don't know, you don't think about "less" and "more." You just feeling whatever right then, and it like, you don't even think, "it's okay, it'll get better." I knew I was getting something, they explained everything, but it was like the words don't make no sense. I couldn't pay attention. I got sick chills, then bad sweats. I couldn't stop yawning even though I wasn't tired, my leg ached and I'd kick the air. My nose be runny like a damn kid.

TODD: Have you heard others describe a similar experience?

JEFF: Damn, I ain't like you! It's not like I'm taking damn notes. [Laughing] No, no one talks about this shit. You think I want to admit this shit? Even to you? I could feel my damn bones under my skin. If I thought about puking I puked, and man that's all I thought about. I kept thinking about eggs and throwing up [laughing]. Eggs! How fucked is that? I'd think about eating—my favorite food is hamburgers, you know, from Checkers, but if I thought about it my throat would get tight and I'd puke.

TODD: Did you know that you were going to come out the other end, since you knew what if felt like from before?

JEFF: No one knows what it's going to be like. You can't remember. I prayed. Fucked up, huh?

TODD: I don't know.

JEFF: You can't hear or see straight, your arms feel too long and your body itches from inside. You can't make a damn fist. You want to bite something, but it hurts to move your mouth. You think shit and your mouth won't move to say the shit you just thought. But after a couple days, the drugs start to do they thing. You forget that you pissed yourself the day before. And you're like, "I'm okay."

TODD: Is it easier to stay on the medication and off other drugs with the experience fresh in your mind?

JEFF: No. That doesn't do it. You go from using, feeling fine, knowing things are fucked, but feeling even. I could work. I'm not going to lie. If I wasn't high all the time I'd be slingin' drugs now. I'm out there, selling, keeping my shit straight. But when you're high, nobody lets you touch nothing. You using not selling. And it's a good thing. I mean, the count be wrong, you use from your stash, someone beat your ass—you get killed, for real. I know it when I stopped using. I could feel it in my stomach. And I was like, "today the day." . . .

But changing from not using to using . . . I don't even know when it happened. You don't feel that. I mean, you know it cause you like, "Hmm . . . I just put some shit in my body," but it's not like something big happens. You feel the shit leaving your body! For real! But coming in is like normal, you don't notice.

TODD: So now you're straight?

JEFF: No, man, I'm going to stay on the "bupe" [buprenorphine] until I get straight. I'm a drug addict, fuck it, but not for long. Fuck all the NA [Narcotics Anonymous] bullshit, all the "hi-my-name-is" bullshit. "Hi, my name is 'fuck you'" [laughing]. I'll get straight, and never see this place again.

TODD: So "bupe" feels like you're still on something?

JEFF: Yeah, I mean, you feel it, sort of, but the main thing is you know you on something.

Jeff offered a description of withdrawal that exceeded a simple recounting of the process itself. His insight regarding substances entering and leaving the body, like a force or possession, was uncanny. Yet there were things that could not be described, which he talked around in order to locate what he felt ("not like being shot," "not like getting your ass beat"). At times he would grab his arm or leg or stomach to show where he hurt. He tugged at his shirt and his skin.

But it is the point of transition that seemed to counter the standard narrative of induction to drug use and then withdrawal. The moment was corporally vague, even if he was conscious of that moment, putting substances "in his body." He said that he knew when the substances "left" his body because of the pain and discomfort, however this wouldn't account for the continuation of buprenorphine used as a replacement therapy and seen as still "being on something." Jeff felt addiction in two ways. First, he knew that his addiction cut him off from work, namely selling drugs. And second, he only "felt" his addiction in the process of withdrawal, when he was moving out of it.

Jeff was forceful when he described "getting straight." He was using Suboxone to help in the process, and recognized how it had helped him in the situation of withdrawal, but it was not imagined as a long-term process (or one that had an undefined end). As I will discuss in the final chapter, Jeff did stop using heroin and other opiates, including buprenorphine. He dropped out of treatment and stopped going to outpatient counseling. He returned to his former occupation, selling drugs on Baltimore's west side. The transition from "addicted" to "straight" brought with it an end to our relationship. Eventually, Jeff's successful weaning from drug dependency allowed him to return to the dangerous economy of the drug trade.

A FAILED ARTIST

I could never shake the image of Francis Bacon's *Three Studies for Figures on a Bed* (1972) from my thoughts when I considered how Jeff described his experience of withdrawal. The image of a body (bodies) writhing on a mattress was too powerful—perhaps a preoccupation with the painting left over from my own former incarnation as a painter. Its circumscribed incompleteness—its visceral-ness—was overwhelming and telling.

Bacon took the human form and made it grotesque and athletic, but never fully formed. He kept these "becoming bodies" in a circumscribed space (sometimes an area drawn on the floor within the painting, or at other times in a box that seemed to float midair around his figures). They could be incomplete and evolving but they were always contained. I take this struggle to contain the figure as it evolves and acquires (or rejects) form as a profoundly ethnographic problem. It is only too obvious to suggest that there is no way to recount all the turns in treatment inside and outside of the clinic. The coherence of the individual accounts, following Goldstein and Foucault, is aimed at making meaning of the facts as they are seen and heard. Not every conversation referred back to drug use or its treatment. The parts of the stories gathered during interviews at the clinic and during visits to homes constituted an assemblage of patienthood where therapeutic intentions joined with social and corporeal circumstance. The temporality of retelling tracked back and forth across situations in the present, those recalled from the past, and those projected into a future. The ethnographic accounts provided outlines of *Figures* (in Deleuze's sense), filled in by some details, the absence and twisting of facts, concealments, and contortions of facts over time. The renderings contrast the assumption that adolescents fall into two distinct categories of pharmaceutically mediated experience: success or failure. The assemblage, here, folds together adolescents who are not model patients but who model (or perform) adherence to the medication, as well as those who refuse adherence and yet become drug free. Both ethnographic and clinical representations of treatment that begin from the point of "successful outcomes" or "failed outcomes" have the danger of offering an image of coherence for adolescents under treatment that runs counter to their experiences with the therapy. Ty, Devon, Heather, and Jeff each painted individual pictures and provided the lines giving contour to experience in their own ways, and creating—to return to Bachelard—the world anew.

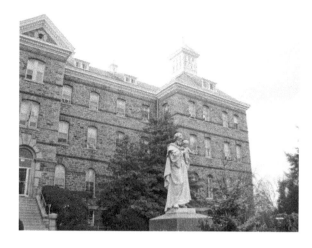

Fig. 1. Main treatment center entrance, front view of the former monastery.

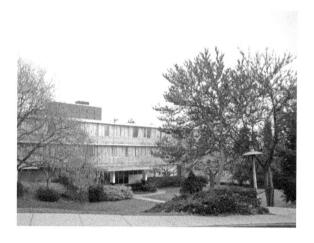

Fig. 2. Residential hall, adjacent to the treatment center entrance.

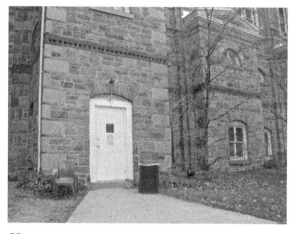

Fig. 3. Staff smoking-break area.

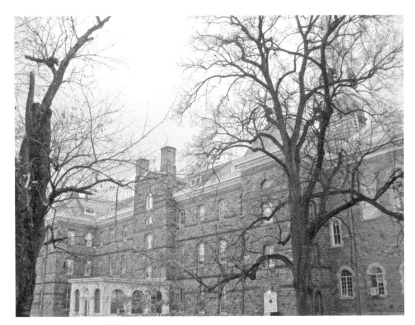

Fig. 4. Rear view of the treatment center.

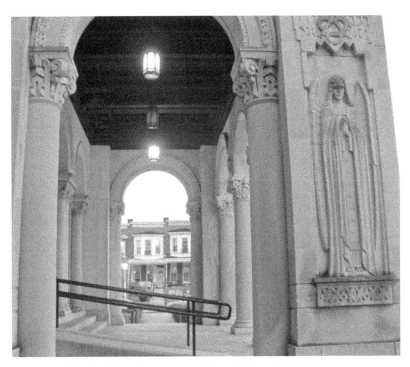

Fig. 5. Neighborhood row houses seen through the cathedral entrance.

3 / APPROPRIATIONS OF CARE

I N THIS CHAPTER, I EXAMINE THE MOVE OF OPIATE DEPENDENCY TREAT-
ment from specialized treatment facilities to office-based settings not only
as a change in clinical geography but as a change that forces a reimagining
of care in relation to therapeutic offerings *between* institutions and *within* the
scope of individual expectations placed on addiction treatment. Through my
interactions with one adolescent, Laura, I hope to provide a small window
onto the values assigned to pharmacotherapy and care, inside and outside
dedicated treatment environments.

CHOICE AND CARE

How does *choice* relate to *care* under the signs of treatment and addiction?
Adolescents abusing drugs make choices that result in very real harm. As
one clinician was fond of telling me, "Kids are very good at making very
bad decisions." But in the case of addiction, the nature of "choice" or "decision making" is not so transparent. Does one decide to become dependent
on substances that put one in harms way—as a misguided pursuit of pleasure or disregard for oneself? On the one hand, it is naive to assume adolescents make whatever decisions they like about drug use and therapy without
regard for the costs. The consequences of addiction were real and felt. On
the other, it is risky to assume that adolescents do not make conscious and
very definitive choices about their drug use and participation in therapy. The
issue is, in part, about the structural conditions and personal circumstances
that limit or constrain—but also sometimes open—choice and agency. Nevertheless, there is some conception of free will and self-determination at
work in relation to the care of oneself with addiction and treatment that
requires appraisal. How do we regard "bad decisions" that may lead to harm

(such as exposure to interpersonal violence, exposure to disease, a loss of self) that sometimes, paradoxically, appear as expressions of self-care?

LAURA

Laura was introduced to me by a clinical staff member at the residential treatment center at an early point in my research. She was not someone who came from a particularly difficult social and family environment, at least not one that was outwardly obvious compared to the other adolescents I followed. Her parents were not members of the "working poor" like so many of the adolescents referred to me, but rather had all the characteristics of the disappearing middle class. Laura's history with opiate abuse, however, was not dissimilar to the other adolescents in residential treatment. By the age of sixteen she had already been using prescription opiates regularly for two years. She started using with a boyfriend, and then continued using without interruption until her parents "forced" her into treatment "against her will"—"kicking and screaming" (to quote her mother).

Laura had been admitted to the treatment center one time prior to the time I met her. Between her previous and present admission, she had seen a private physician in Baltimore who prescribed Suboxone to treat her dependency. According to her account, the treatment was not at all successful:

> You have to understand something. Maybe it's just me, but I don't think you can just give someone a pill and expect everything to be fine. Pills are the problem! At least my problem . . . I'm *really* good at taking pills [laughing]. I took it [Suboxone], but I kept using [other drugs]. I'd come in for more "bupe" [buprenorphine] and the doctor would be all, "You're still using. Why? Isn't the treatment working?" And I was like, "Of course I am, why not?" When there's nobody paying attention, I kinda felt like I could do whatever. He was a nice guy and all, but I was like, whatever.

I asked Laura about her suggestion that people couldn't be trusted to follow a physician's orders about medication—something that was a motif in our conversations at the treatment center:

TODD: Is it something specific to Suboxone, or are you saying that
nobody can be trusted with any pill?

LAURA: No, I mean, it's just with this drug. Actually, no, I mean it about
every drug. People don't take antibiotics like they're supposed to.
Why do you think my parents have about ten different half-empty
prescription bottles in the cabinet? You take something until you feel
better. Period. And when I'm using, how I feel is all that matters to
me, even if it pisses everybody off.

TODD: So you only took Suboxone until you felt better, then you
stopped taking it?

LAURA: No, I kept taking it. Tastes like a penny under your tongue,
but I kept taking it. I didn't see a reason to stop. But I didn't see any
reason to stop taking other things, too.

What is odd about the conversation I had with Laura, regarding her experience with the private physician, is that she could easily have repeated the pattern of continued abuse of prescription opiates while in residential and outpatient care (others had, and were). But this wasn't the case. She stuck with Suboxone, and offered every indication that she planned to continue with her treatment without using other drugs while at the residential center. "I'm part of something here," she told me. But what exactly she was "part of" remained unclear.

The more I spoke with her throughout her time in treatment, the more the connectedness she had with other adolescents at the center became increasingly clear. Her comportment changed over weeks in residential treatment. She picked up forms of speech that were not present early in our conversations. She used terms like "drug of choice" and "my history of abuse," phrases so many of the other adolescents deployed effortlessly after countless group therapy sessions. And when it was time for her to be discharged into intensive outpatient treatment, she was genuinely sad to leave. I followed her around as she hugged residential staff and other adolescents with whom she'd become close during her time at the center—who were numerous. Her departure was hopeful, but for her part, shot through with sadness.

I continued to speak with Laura during her outpatient visits to the treatment center. She expressed a longing to come back, to be readmitted. When I asked what her plans were (for school, for work, when she planned to take driver's training) she was vague. Eventually, she stopped coming to outpatient treatment. When I spoke with her mother, she told me that Laura had resumed treatment with the same private physician.

THE LIMITS OF CONTROL

Two days before I ended my time at the treatment center, Laura was readmitted. She was not withdrawn or strung out. She actually appeared joyful, if a little worse for wear. When I asked her why she came back, she provided a simple answer: "I missed this place."

While Laura was at the treatment center, she was a model patient. "She's wonderful," one of the caseworkers told me, "I'll never understand why she keeps returning to us. If she's behaving the same way when she's referred out, she should have no problems." Laura would adhere to the psychosocial and pharmaceutical therapy while in the treatment center, but as soon as she lacked whatever structure, whatever sense of attachment she had there, things fell apart. She told me: "When I'm here, on the inside, it's not the same as when I'm on the outside. There's nothing the same about being treated with the same thing."

Laura expressed a strong desire to be in treatment, specifically treatment at the residential center. Laura's mother recognized this desire. "She likes it here too much. But we hate it," she told me during a family visit on Laura's second admission into treatment. "We feel like we're abandoning her to this place," her mother said as Laura's father nodded strongly. She continued:

We want her to make good decisions, and we try to give her the space to do that at home. We really make little demand on her. She can go to school, be with her friends. She's our only child and we treat her that way. She's popular! I mean, at her school, too. We don't like the influence here. The stories she tells us about the other kids make my hair stand on end. Sexual abuse, rape, HIV—that's not our Laura—and still she identifies with these kids. I'm sure they're good kids, but you know, we worry. We really try our best. Laura's never even been paddled!

[Laura's father interjects, "Christ, no!"] Her father and I have never touched drugs—I hate taking medications of any kind, even when I'm sick—how does she even get them we ask?

Laura's parents were insistent on their refusal to be "controlling," which they saw as just "inviting kids to act out." But as Laura describes her relationship with her parents, she explains that she is "kind of expected to fuck up." Moreover, Laura wanted the space (outside of the home) to make her own, "messy" decisions. Despite the highly orchestrated routines in the residential treatment center—routines that many of the other adolescents felt were too restrictive and that they actively resisted—and however contradictorily, Laura saw "being on her own," in treatment, as offering a degree of freedom not afforded at home. The residential treatment center, "with all its rules," was still a space where she could be an "adult," where she could decide whether to "fuck up or not fuck up." Laura regarded home (and her continued treatment with the private physician) as a place where she was left with no choice but to make bad decisions.

THE LOGIC OF CARE

In her book, *The Logic of Care: Health and the Problem of Patient Choice,* Annemarie Mol addresses patient autonomy and the pursuit of health as a contest between logics of care and logics of choice.[1] Individual choice, and, more importantly for Mol, the acknowledgment that individuals deserve to be *heard* in the medical encounter, is affirmed as a precondition of the therapeutic process. The argument Mol develops—one that is of great importance—is that, under the banner of medical consumerism, "choice" is equated with a vague desire to attain "the good life." She writes, "in care practices our minds are called upon, not our desires." And yet, given the realities of illness and disorder, care is not always rational: "our desires may not be rational, but, or so logic of care has it, neither are our minds. Instead, they are full of gaps, contradictions, and obsessions."[2] Mol's distinction between *care* and *choice* separates facts from values—leaving the *act* and *conditions* of care and caregiving in a bind of irrationality where many of us are, in fact, complicit.[3]

In Mol's thesis we find a struggle to disentangle oneself from the collective. Furthermore, she raises interesting and difficult questions about the limits and values applied to conceptualizations of *self-care*. As an object of anthropological inquiry, one need only look as far as Arthur Frank's attempts to reconcile the concealment necessary "to take care of ourselves" with the desire to secure meaning in the "confession" or "narration" of disorder.[4] In the third volume of *The History of Sexuality*, we find Michel Foucault's conception of "the care of the self."[5] "Self care," cultivating or "taking care of oneself," renews the stakes of the individual—but one thing that remains a struggle in the specific case is how activities in the therapeutic process (of treating opiate dependency) seem to blur the conditions necessary for *self care* and *care* as an ethical relationship with others—something echoed in various ways in the works of Ludwig Wittgenstein, Stanley Cavell, Emmanuel Levinas, and others[6]—and moreover, how these relationships are articulated through sets of therapeutic practices and the not-so-transparent act of caring for another individual. Carol Gilligan's "ethics of care" does, in part, offer a design—one not limited to abstract principles of political economy or justice.[7] Care, in Gilligan's work, renews value in social activities oriented toward the care of others, while still accounting for the complicated moral texture of human relations—a concern taken up by Michel Foucault as well.[8] The attempt to redefine relations of dependence constitutes a starting point for an "ethics of care," or at least one that reformulates theories of justice on the basis of a political anthropology, seeking to account for the relational constitution of moral agents.[9]

"Care" as the *result* of medical intervention would have to account for both the object (the pill) as well as the actions that go into making objects vehicles for therapy (psychosocial therapy, physician orders, and so on). Céline Lefève has recently argued that medical techniques, including in their materiality, can be thought of as containing the features of care.[10] Yet the meanings attached to a statement like "caring for someone" seem very close to the practical ideal of therapeutic intervention. What is interesting here is that *care/caring* and *therapeutics* become theoretically (practically) difficult to distinguish—which is fine, but this would require us to mobilize in an intense way both the question of care *and* the question of therapeutics. Care, it seems, is situated somewhere between an *event* or *moment* and a set of conditions (institutional, intersubjective) which make its offering possible. These *conditions* would have to include constrained agency, the singular problems of patienthood, the biomedical environment, and a complicated set of formal and informal institutional arrangements—making *the logic of care* deeply bound up with an administrative logic of therapeutics, acting as a kind of connective tissue between the self as an agent of her therapy (but where the direction of therapy could go wildly off track) and therapeutics— as well as a link between clinical environments and the patients that enter these spaces.

NEW GEOGRAPHIES

The Drug Addiction Treatment Act allowed buprenorphine to be prescribed for treatment outside highly monitored clinical environments, opening a new therapeutic space.[11] When the drugs Reckitt Benckiser Pharmaceuticals developed were approved in October 2002, private office-based treatment of opiate dependency became a clinical reality.[12] The rescheduling of buprenorphine and the FDA approval of the new drugs marked a victory for the drug company and for advocates of more comprehensive addiction treatment. However, along with a growing optimism, concerns about prescription opioid abuse and new populations of opiate abusers (namely adolescents experimenting with prescription painkillers, as well as older adults with no prior history of opiate abuse whose dependency followed the treatment of chronic or postoperative pain) began to take shape.[13]

At first glance the story of buprenorphine seems analogous to that of methadone thirty years earlier. And much like methadone, the promise of buprenorphine as an effective drug for treating opiate dependency has slowly begun to erode from (or at least has become bound up with) anxieties about drug diversion and abuse.[14] There are, however, a number of significant differences in the two cases. On a pharmacological level, buprenorphine is far less likely to produce negative side effects such as respiratory distress than methadone, making the management of treatment with pharmacotherapy much safer and more therapeutically desirable than any previous replacement therapy. The greatest distinction, however, is found in the treatment setting itself. Unlike methadone, buprenorphine is available outside highly monitored, specialized treatment environments. Private physicians, after completing some brief training modules through the Substance Abuse and Mental Health Services Administration (SAMHSA), can prescribe buprenorphine in private, office-based settings on an outpatient basis. Rather than referring patients to specialized addiction-treatment services, suddenly the prescribing physician has the capacity to use individual judgment in offering treatment, with the change constituting an expanded clinical role.[15] And yet, or rather despite this migration, buprenorphine remains stuck between two competing narratives: one of *sameness*—reproducing concerns regarding individual risk and public threat—and one of *difference*—a narrative that attempts to secure new hope that the drug and its treatment modality will allow clinicians to more effectively chip away at the problems of addiction. Not only do these sentiments echo through public and professional discourse, they also reverberate through discussions between physicians, family members, and patients regarding stated expectations as they come to terms with treatment.

The move from highly monitored treatment facilities to private, office-based outpatient settings changed not only the space in which treatment occurs, but also how addiction treatment has come to be conceptualized.[16] While there are tremendous benefits associated with the wider availability of pharmaceuticals for treatment of dependency, there is also a widening gap between public and private spheres—as well as between the group and the individual.[17] My discussions with physicians in both private settings and within dedicated in-patient drug treatment facilities suggest the gap is not so much (or not *just*) socioeconomic (separating those who can afford private treatment and those who cannot), but is found in the increasing distance in the way treatment is imagined by physicians, patients, and families.

Laura's family could afford private treatment, although not without some financial burden. But the issue, according to Laura's father, was not at all financial in nature. Laura's father was a veteran of the Gulf War, where he served as a sergeant. After the war, he went to technical school and began working as a maintenance supervisor in a Veteran's Administration (VA) hospital. "You wouldn't believe the things these kids have to deal with coming back from Iraq and Afghanistan," he told me during a visit to Laura's home. "The drugs, the limb loss, the hopelessness. I served in the same theater and I can't relate to them at all." Laura's father expressed great concern about these returning men and women "getting lost in the system." "They sort of get dependent on the military and then the VA. I was lucky and I'm thankful to have a better future for serving, but these kids . . . god."

Laura's father was clear that he did not want Laura to get lost in a system that "robs kids of a future." His ability to make a professional career, to "have a better future," was directly linked to his desire to keep Laura out of residential treatment. "I see the VA and [name of the center] as part of the same system," he said. "I would never forgive myself if I gave her up to it." It is not so much that class or socioeconomic conditions create a distance between public and private treatment, but it is the meaning (for Laura's father) attached to each of these places that required distancing—one associated with "the system" and one associated with care and the promise of a better future.

FEAR AND PROMISE

The treatment of opiate dependency with other opiates is not simply substitution. The pharmacokinetic properties of substances are only one point along the therapeutic register where each comes to operate.[18] Not all opioids are the same (pharmacologically) and not all opioids have been received in the same way (clinically, socially, politically). The analgesic properties of morphine, methadone, and heroin were each at different times in their respective histories seen to have therapeutic value. Perhaps the most recent example demonstrating the complicated way therapeutic value is understood can be found in the controversy regarding the use of heroin as a replacement therapy for opiate abuse in parts of Europe.[19] The "practicality" and effectiveness of a drug in the clinical context is not enough to quiet social concern about misuse—and not enough to erase its historical associations. Even in environments where the management of therapy is highly monitored, opiates remain troubling when they reside at the center of treatment.[20] Nevertheless, historical transformations and local contexts fail to explain how buprenorphine has made such an impact on the reconceptualization of dependency treatment, while still retaining a vague aura of threat that cannot be reconciled against the way treatment is actually on offer.

When a brief article appeared in *The New England Journal of Medicine* announcing the approval of buprenorphine for office-based treatment of opiate dependency, it included a promise that buprenorphine would not become a substitute drug of abuse as methadone had become.[21] Buprenorphine offered a pharmacologically "finer tuned" replacement therapy.[22] But even with a new treatment at the disposal of a wider range of clinicians, the public health concern about the large number of opiate-addicted people not currently being treated for dependency persisted.[23] The clinical presentation of a patient with opioid dependence is not new in the context of private office-based treatment; what is new is the ability to treat patients for drug dependency in this setting.[24]

NO LONGER SPECIAL

"It's so important that we have these drugs. You wouldn't believe how great the problem of dependency is," a young physician working in a private behavioral health center told me:

> It's not like the problem is new—my god, what is? But "bupe" is *novel* because you can no longer think about addiction without thinking about what's in your [pharmacological] arsenal to fight it, and not just because you're in addiction medicine. Here's a new weapon, and it makes addiction new. Do you get my meaning? It's impossible to think about drug dependency without thinking about the intervention at the same time. At least for me . . .

He went on to explain that there is "no one approach" for office-based treatment, just as there is no one approach for formal in-patient dependency treatment:

> Yes, I completed the SAMHSA training, but the modules tend to muddle clinical practice. On one side, you're given training in diagnosing dependency and abuse for non-specialists, like DSM-lite [referring to the *Diagnostic and Statistical Manual of Mental Disorders: DSM-IV-TR*]. And on the other side, you're given a set of tools for monitoring progress and recording where the pills are going. But it's the middle part, the treatment, that isn't well defined—which I suppose is good, since they trust our judgment as physicians. I imagine if you spoke with another hundred physicians you'd find a hundred different approaches to managing treatment.

I did interview over a hundred other physicians, mostly by phone. It was hard to characterize their perspectives on treatment as singular, other than that it was a positive transformation. The availability of buprenorphine in office-based settings was adopted in various ways from the beginning.[25] The experiment in the late 1990s to treat opiate dependency with methadone in primary care settings rather than methadone clinics was seen as completely different by the physicians I spoke with.[26] "You can't even begin to compare," an internist working in a primary care clinic serving low-income families in southwest Baltimore told me:

> I was one of the docs who was part of this [move toward clinic-based methadone treatment]. We could have decorated the lobby with all the red tape I went through [laughing]. It was a disaster. It certainly didn't lessen the stigma of methadone . . . it just put a spotlight on it. I'm treating upwards of twenty patients with "bupe" and I've not encountered any problem. It really hasn't changed much administratively.

I was interested in whether or not the two approaches (inpatient treatment and office-based treatment) were perceived to work differently, or one better than the other.[27] "Yes and no," a psychiatrist specializing in addiction medicine told me at the residential treatment center:

> Psychosocial therapy is a pretty important addition to the medication, but the drugs and dosages are largely the same in either, and monitoring is pretty much the same. We do directly observed therapy in the study, but as soon as the switch happens to outpatient treatment, we trust that they're still following their scripts [prescriptions]. So it's pretty much the same in private treatment.

A question that is difficult to answer from the perspective of the individual clinician, however, is whether or not the treatment is actually reaching new populations.[28] The Baltimore Health Commissioner, Dr. Joshua M. Sharfstein, fought to expand treatment services through the "Baltimore Buprenorphine Initiative" in 2006. The expansion made buprenorphine the front line treatment of opiate addiction in the city.[29] An early problem faced by the initiative, however, was finding physicians to become certified to prescribe. Physicians did complete mandatory reporting when using buprenorphine, but it was unclear to what extent buprenorphine was systematically adopted in both public and private settings.[30] Something that remained a lingering concern (for clinicians and for the news media) had to do with changes in the *appearance* of treatment between public and private therapeutic environments, as well as who was *doing the looking*.[31] The physicians I spoke with who worked in private, office-based settings shared sentiments regarding treatment similar to those of physicians working in inpatient treatment settings. And yet a sharper distinction between these clinical environments emerges as patients pass through both settings at different points in their therapeutic careers.

CARE SEEN AND UNSEEN

"I'm glad I made it back," Laura told me on her return to the residential treatment center, "I worked *hard* to get back here [smiling]." In Laura's case it's unclear if her affinity for the treatment center was the reason why her time is treatment was so "successful" compared with her time in private treatment. It seems wrong to assign intentions that don't account for the social worlds in which she was enmeshed outside the residential treatment center. But Laura's story does begin to work against an assumption that office-based treatment is an equivalent treatment environment, or that individualized treatment in these settings necessarily leads to better outcomes. "I'm just happy if people can get help wherever they can find it," one of the clinicians at the treatment center told me, "Christ, whatever works."

In Laura's case, there is a complicated set of objects and actors put into place to find out "what works"—or, to use Annemarie Mol's terminology, there is a mix of facts and values at work in the choice of a care environment. But what Laura found to "work" is different from what Laura's parents envisaged. The conditions of care—allowing freedom at home, not controlling, keeping Laura out of the system—were conceptualized in ways opposed to how Laura imagined independence, and indeed the process of recovery. Laura's desire to possess "messy" agency—to make her own choices—remains stuck in a morass of lived experience that demands consideration of what happens "outside" and "inside" treatment. Unfortunately, in the case of addiction, learning from one's mistakes may have disastrous consequences.

Laura made the *choice* to be in residential treatment rather than to remain in a private setting "on the outside." But what kind of choice is this? Can it be called *self-care*? Or even a form of decision making that follows some kind of medico-consumer logic? In the end, we are left with logics of choice and logics of care that conform to institutional and therapeutic demand, and imaginations of care and the desire for caregiving (in pharmacotherapy, in the family, in place—in simply *being there* at the treatment center) as therapy is offered in the clinic and other spaces. And lastly, we are left with complicated assessments of individual behaviors that refuse easy attributions of individual agency.

4 / THERAPY AND REASON

I N DECEMBER 2007, *THE BALTIMORE SUN* PUBLISHED A SERIES OF FEA-
ture articles profiling the relatively recent use of buprenorphine to treat
opiate addiction in Baltimore.[1] The articles spanned the use of the drug in
sub-Saharan Africa, France, and a number of cities in the United States in
order to contextualize the local impact of the treatment. In addition to offering a short history of the drug and its implementation, *The Baltimore Sun*
reported that the police had seized 24 and a half buprenorphine "pills" from
a man selling them along Pennsylvania Avenue on Baltimore's west side.
Self-medication and drug diversion were subjects discussed by the reporters
in anonymous "street interviews" conducted throughout the city. The basic
narrative of the articles was clear: the therapy was clinically promising but
suffered from widespread abuse and misuse. The main concern centered on
new markets for the illegal sale of the drug toward non-therapeutic ends:

> Buprenorphine's wide availability is starting to create some of the prob-
> lems it was meant to solve. An investigation by *The Sun* has found that
> patients are selling their prescriptions illegally, creating a new drug of
> abuse that some people are injecting to get high.[2]

A few days after *The Baltimore Sun* ran the stories, the *City Paper*, a local
alternative weekly, ran a similar story, echoing claims of growing abuse in
Maryland.[3] Indeed, there were many physicians in Maryland prescribing
the drug to treat opiate-dependent patients—at the time, there were slightly
more than 400 doctors signed up to prescribe buprenorphine and the prescription volume was the seventh highest in the country.[4] Despite the volume, there were few—if any—physicians in the Baltimore area who reported
grave concern about patients misusing or selling their prescriptions.[5]

RESPONDING IN KIND

The Baltimore Sun articles provoked an immediate response. Rolley E. John-son, vice president for scientific and regulatory affairs of Reckitt Benckiser Pharmaceuticals, wrote an official letter from the pharmaceutical company responding to the characterization and extent of the problem suggested in the reports, emphasizing the company's intentions to thwart continued mis-use.[6] The letter conceded poor surveillance. The company acknowledged incidences of abuse but failed to deepen the discussion of the drug's abuse potential or how prescribing practices and surveillance might be improved. The aim of the letter was to assure a concerned public that everything was being done to prevent abuse. The drug manufacturer avoided a vehement defense of its product, opting instead to maintain a picture of integrity while promising increased scrutiny of existing mechanisms for surveillance.[7]

Dr. Joshua M. Sharfstein, the Baltimore Health Commissioner, was con-siderably less deferential in his response to the articles. In a strongly worded letter to the editor, Sharfstein wrote that the reports worked to "obscure the enormous good that has already come to hundreds of thousands" and ignored the fact that the treatment "saves lives."[8] Even in the face of potential abuse and misuse, the benefits outweighed the problems—and compared histori-cally to the illegal sale and diversion of methadone, buprenorphine's situation paled.[9] Close to the time of the articles, Sharfstein asked the Maryland General Assembly to expand buprenorphine treatment by $5 million. The request was warranted. Only a few months before the publication of the *The Baltimore Sun* articles, the Maryland State Medical Society produced a study in which they found the biggest hurdle related to effective treatment was not misuse and diversion but cost.[10] Nevertheless, the articles appearing in *The Baltimore Sun* continued to generate concern. Only a few days after the first article in the series had been published, the Maryland State Senate called for a probe into the abuse of buprenorphine. The legislators were concerned about misuse of the drug, though they were equally concerned about the misuse of tax dollars to support what seemed like a problematic form of treatment.[11] The claims regarding poor surveillance leading to diversion and the alleged incidences of illegal sale were at the core of the debate. The findings of the Senate probe two months after *The Baltimore Sun* articles first appeared described the prob-lem of abuse as "serious" and "dangerous," and suggested that the problem might be largely due to "negligence" on the part of the medical community.[12]

Apprehension about abuse and diversion of buprenorphine was not a new topic; it was there from the beginning. In 1978, during the time Donald Jasinski and his colleagues were scrutinizing the treatment potential of the analgesic Buprenex, they were also examining the analgesic's abuse potential.[13] They found the potential for abuse—as well as the potential for negative outcomes such as respiratory distress—to be far less than existing treatments, namely the full μ-receptor agonist therapy, methadone. The Substance Abuse and Mental Health Services Administration (SAMHSA) first became aware of "anecdotal" cases of abuse and diversion in December 2005, outlined in a report based on the findings of Food and Drug Administration (FDA) mandated post-marketing surveillance set up by Reckitt Benckiser Pharmaceuticals—post-marketing surveillance that had been in place since 2003.[14] In his oversight of the buprenorphine initiative, Dr. H. Westley Clark, the Director of the Center for Substance Abuse Treatment under SAMHSA, was determined to keep the focus on the therapeutic effects in the treatment of heroin abuse and dependence (understanding drug addiction as a public health problem) and not on potential abuse and diversion.[15] Dr. Charles R. Schuster, a physician who gave congressional testimony in 2002 during the hearings on the drug's approval and a past director of the National Institute on Drug Abuse (NIDA) who conducted clinical trials on the buprenorphine and naloxone combination drug Suboxone, maintained that only a very small percentage of opiate-dependent users have experimented with the drug, based on the collection of national statistics on abuse and diversion.[16] Nevertheless, public concern persisted.

There were those who believed the problem was significant, and that it rested primarily with physicians. Dr. David Fiellin, a Yale professor who directs the Physician Clinical Support System, has proposed that the problem with misuse and diversion of buprenorphine may lie with physicians who practice outside the standards of care.[17] He goes on to suggest that the combination of a lack of active surveillance and practices of overprescribing by physicians obscure the chances of discovering whether patients are selling their prescriptions, or whether patients are crushing and injecting the drugs themselves toward nontherapeutic ends. Despite the fact that physicians are limited in the number of patients they are allowed to treat (currently 100 patients per physician), perceptions that prescribing practices have gone off the rails pervade.[18] In an outline of strategies to reduce misuse and diversion, Reckitt Benckiser Pharmaceuticals planned to train doctors how to improve prescribing practices in order to reduce the abuse of buprenorphine and to increase awareness of the practices of crushing and injecting.[19]

Doug Donovan and Fred Schulte, the two reporters responsible for the December 2007 articles in *The Baltimore Sun*, continued to write on the abuse of buprenorphine in Baltimore throughout 2008. In April, they reported on police seizures and evidence of increasing illegal sales. They associated the increase with a national trend, but argued that Baltimore warranted special attention. Donovan and Schulte described the contents of an internal Baltimore Police Department document that noted that Suboxone was "widely available" on the street, ranging in price from $5 to $10 per pill. The report documented 182 cases of buprenorphine seizures in 2007, and offered anecdotes on the arrest of a 31-year-old woman holding two dozen Suboxone pills and a prescription bottle with a scratched-out label, and a 53-year-old man arrested who possessed "a bottle with an 'obliterated' label containing 38 Suboxone pills and $302 in cash" to support its claims.[20] However, it is unclear how many of these seizures were made from individuals who possessed legal prescriptions. The article ends with a quote from Dr. Elinore F. McCance-Katz, president of the American Academy of Addiction Psychiatry: "We must address this issue of diversion. If this drug is seen as something that is potentially harming the public, we want to get in front of that. As physicians we need to look at this very carefully."[21]

TECHNOLOGIES OF SUSPICION

Many details remain puzzling about *The Baltimore Sun* articles and the reactions they provoked. On all sides, little effort was made to differentiate between the two treatment drugs. Subutex (buprenorphine) and Suboxone (buprenorphine-naloxone, the drug most commonly prescribed in Baltimore) were consistently conflated in the debates. It was "bupe" (as buprenorphine is called in Baltimore) that came to denote both treatment drugs. While both drugs are partial μ-receptor agonists, Suboxone—a combination of buprenorphine and naloxone—is also a partial μ-receptor antagonist, making its abuse by opiate users with long careers of dependence nearly impossible (or at least improbable). Dr. Christopher Welsh of the University of Maryland School of Medicine wrote in a letter to the newspaper that "*The Sun* sensationalizes claims of abuse—no serious addict would seek this drug out for abuse."[22] The ceiling effect provided by naloxone in the drug Suboxone is simply prohibitive. In France, Subutex is the most commonly prescribed treatment and was offered by *The Baltimore Sun* as an example of an analogous experience of growing abuse and diversion.[23] But the frontline treatment in Baltimore is not the same, and the different drugs (Suboxone and Subutex) do not share (pharmacologically) the same "abuse potential."[24] Moreover, the evidence in the articles citing Subutex abuse in the urban United States were drawn almost exclusively from Worcester, Massachusetts, not Baltimore. Lastly, the articles link the epidemic of heroin abuse to the risk for human immunodeficiency virus (HIV) infection through injecting practices—thus creating a very specific picture of the type of abuse (and abuser) imagined. However, there is not one example given of an individual crushing tablets and injecting the drug, or even a combination of drugs. Moreover, the articles failed to distinguish between the problems of heroin addiction and the increasing abuse of prescription painkillers such as Oxycontin.

It is not surprising that the articles failed to address these specific though arguably crucial details. Only so much can be asked of a journalistic account. What is surprising, however, is that nowhere do we find detailed arguments offered in response to what can only be described as damning indictments of the therapy. The articles make it seem as though the treatment of opiate dependence using buprenorphine offers little more than new possibilities for abuse requiring attenuation. But how accurate is the perspective? Where does it find its empirical ground? Even a Baltimore City Grand Jury found that the abuse and diversion of buprenorphine was minor despite the fact that the problems associated with addiction were so great. The jury suggested that efforts should be made to significantly increase treatment offerings in the city.[25] In the face of overwhelming evidence suggesting the benefits of the treatment, *The Baltimore Sun* still fomented public concern. As Joshua Sharfstein and Peter Luongo, the Maryland State Director of Alcohol and Drug Abuse Administration, point out, *The Baltimore Sun* did so, successfully, without addressing the larger social and economic dilemmas associated with drug abuse, without citing interviews with anyone in Baltimore whose primary problem was buprenorphine abuse, and through the citation of unnamed critics. In the letters to the editor responding to the first series of feature articles, Diana Morris, Director of the Open Society Institute-Baltimore, wrote that *The Baltimore Sun*'s characterization "distorts the picture of a promising therapy, with no focus on high social costs."[26]

OTHER PEOPLE'S PROBLEMS

How does the potential for individual misuse lead to fears of new or renewed forms of public harm? The issue is not whether the pharmaceutical is or has ever been used nontherapeutically, rather, *the issue is how a conception of therapy and therapeutics against abuse is itself imagined*, and how categories of *licit* therapeutic opiate use and *illicit* nontherapeutic uses become unstable. *The Baltimore Sun*'s reporting represented the public consumption of private danger as a shift away from individual behavioral risk and toward a generalized anxiety regarding the collapse of regulation and the threat of unchecked abuse under the sign of medical expedience.[27] The anthropological concern—at least here—is not about new forms of drug abuse, but is instead on the way drug-addicted people are viewed and imagined in relation to therapy, and how that imagining often does not match individual experience.[28] What is most troubling in the media account of "medication leaking" is the failure to recognize that opiate-dependant individuals under treatment with replacement therapy might actually be using other opiates simultaneously.[29] To put the question simply, *Can medicine absorb the individual as both addict and patient?*[30]

A complex calculus is at work in negotiating harm, risk, and danger in relation to a new therapy—including concerns about potential misuse, abuse, and the possibility that new underground markets of illicit use will take hold. Situated within this complexity is a persistent question: *What happens when patients are thought to be working against a given therapy*? And how then is noncompliance factored into (or seen to depart from) clinical reasoning? As Jeremy Greene has argued in an essay on the nomenclature of noncompliance, or what he calls *therapeutic infidelities*, ideas about noncompliance are not only about patients doing (or not doing) what they are told by physicians; they are ways of managing the uncertainty of therapy itself.[31] Noncompliance implies a very clear idea of how and why interventions, in this case, pharmacological interventions, are effective and how they should be properly used—and how the risk of misuse is managed.[32]

However, there remains a lived reality outside the laboratory or the clinic, one where individuals make choices beyond the scope intended by medicine, and where not only drugs but also forms of reasoning seem to be diverted.

CEDRIC AND MEGAN

While following adolescents inside and outside the clinic, I spent a considerable amount of time with a young couple, Cedric and Megan. Their lives (together and individually) over the period I knew them wove (and swerved) in and out of residential drug-dependency treatment and various other clinical environments, most notably short-term psychiatric hospitalizations. Through their stories, the processes and logics of self-medication that bind a sense of social, bodily, and intimate security become clear—while also exposing the basis for social and medical concerns regarding the danger of drug misuse for the individual.

Cedric and Megan were assigned different designations of patienthood at different times, determined largely by the environments through which they passed. But it was the designation of drug-dependent person that held constant meaning. Dependency for both Cedric and Megan was not only a label but something felt internally: dependency was an ache and a hurt and a pleasure and a bodily habit—but also something that they believed needed intervention externally.

I followed Megan and Cedric, who were both sixteen years old at the time I met them, from inpatient drug treatment, through outpatient treatment, and into Cedric's mother's house where they both were living—which was a period of about eighteen months altogether.

DIVERTING DRUGS AND REASON

I was surprised that the photo on the cover of the church program from Cedric's brother's funeral, placed next to a small collection of silk flowers on the coffee table, looked so much like Cedric himself. My gaze lingered a little too long on the photograph as I sat deeply in an oversized couch across from Cedric and Megan in Cedric's mother's living room. "My Moms said we were like twins she had two years apart." I smiled, though the image was uncanny—

more like an object from a not so distant future impinging on the present. Another teenager had stabbed Cedric's brother to death during an argument about stolen drugs—drugs allegedly stolen by Cedric's brother (who was a low-level dealer) from a main stash to support his own habit. Cedric gave some indication that he knew the boy who had stabbed his brother, but his description lacked a current of anger or judgment. "You looking at what I ain't, or ain't going to . . ." His words trailed off as though he had lost the thread of his thought, hoping to turn attention elsewhere. Cedric had been using prescription painkillers and heroin (smoking and snorting, although he insisted that he never shot heroin intravenously) for at least three years, and Megan for considerably less time. Cedric had only been in residential treatment once, at the time I met him. After an arrest for assault he had been ordered into treatment instead of being sent to a juvenile criminal facility.

By all accounts, he was successful during his time in the treatment center. He had minimal withdrawal symptoms and reported less craving during his stay. He was "diligent" (to borrow a word from one of the clinical staff when I discussed Cedric with her). He continued (now with Megan, also a treatment center patient) to see the clinical staff once every few weeks for a supply of pills, and attended outpatient group therapy based loosely on the Narcotics Anonymous twelve-step model, but tailored for adolescents and young adults.

Cedric was a tall, lanky teenager with a deeply rutted face that seemed too old for his body. He wore the same green and yellow oversized warm-up suit for months on end, and given his slight frame it was not hard to imagine his body swimming beneath the clothes. His eyes were always heavy during our conversations, something I mistook for boredom, only to realize later that it was part affect and part exhaustion. Cedric was exhausted by the simplest tasks. He would slowly peel himself off the couch when his mother called to him from another room. Cedric acted very much like an adult, a middle-aged man, though his mother called him "baby" and made him "do chores" every day. I resisted the urge to attribute his fatigue to some underlying medical condition, and at times would forget that his slow movements were also the effects of a steady accumulation of drugs in his system.

Cedric looked remarkably changed from the Polaroid that was stapled to his research study file, taken a year before. He was older, thinner, and his features were more intense. In the photograph taken three days into his hospitalization (detoxification) at the treatment center, his eyes float, as though they are trying to maintain a focus on something, anything. His hair is partially braided, with the combed-out half extending outside of the frame of the photograph. It wasn't long after his hospitalization that he met Megan through a mutual friend.

Megan was thin, blonde, and fragile in her appearance. She shared Cedric's weathered look, and though she still passed as a young girl, her hands were rough and covered with healed-over scars from cigarette burns. She had been in treatment several times, and had dropped out only to reenroll in the clinical trial, twice. She eventually dropped out altogether after expressing some vague paranoia that she was being "dosed" by the research staff. "I'm not a chimp," she told me between long drags off her cigarette while cradling her McDonald's coffee.

Megan's distrust of the treatment staff did not stop her from attempting to treat her own addiction. Cedric and Megan described in great detail how they were managing their dependency on opiates: "We just cut a little, snort a little [heroin] and then take the 'bupe' pill [Suboxone]." Megan added: "Sometimes, a little OC [Oxycontin] sometimes, you know, to balance." Cedric was emphatic every time I wanted to discuss their therapeutic regime: "It just like in group, you know, cut back a little, and a little more, and bad days less, and some day, you know, cured." They had indeed been reducing the amounts and proportions throughout. A small spiral notebook was produced as evidence. "We keep a chart."

Cedric's statement is ironic, but this is precisely the point. It was a clinical record of a closely self-monitored process of replacement therapy. Of course, when it came to heroin, the *stability* [purity] of each dose varied—wildly—and "tapering" was more akin to tiny increments, but the rationale was the same—a simulacrum of clinical reasoning.[33] Moreover, for Cedric and Megan there was a picture of a future, one free of dependency. Somehow that future was not as potent as the present moment—one filled with an attitude of success and the resistance to a shared fate of his "twin" brother.

When I would see Cedric on his own, which happened rarely, he would tell me of his suspicion that Megan was using heroin besides the times the two of them would use together. Megan and Cedric would often hang out with Wayne, a close friend of Cedric's who was a few years older, and someone whose affection for Megan was clear. Megan would catch rides with Wayne to her own mother's house to collect clothes, and occasionally money and food, but mainly she would go to visit her younger siblings. I never brought the subject up, but I was curious why Cedric would elect to stay at his own house during these times rather than ride to Megan's house with Wayne and Megan.

"If we'd just stay with the 'rehab,' we'll be fine," Cedric told me, implying that this was not happening with Megan. Strangely, when I would go with Megan to get food at the corner store after the outpatient treatment meetings at the clinic, she shared the same suspicions about Cedric. "The motherfucker doesn't think I can count," she barked, referring to the number of pills remaining between times that they used together. It was only once that she offered a window into the deep anxiety and jealousy over Cedric's relationship with Wayne. She had borrowed my cell phone, called Cedric, and screamed "Get a fucking room" into the phone—shoving it back into my hand, on the verge of tears.

The "chart" Cedric and Megan kept was some means of monitoring one another, however imperfectly. The chart was *clinical* in the strictest sense, but it was also *social* and *intimate*: a document of multiple fidelities, including *therapeutic fidelity*, to reverse Jeremy Greene's formulation. So what are the issues? Here is a case of self-medication, noncompliance, and patterns of substance abuse seen and unseen. So how do we begin to truly contend with the lived realities of *therapeutics*? It's not enough to say that Cedric and Megan are mirroring clinical reasoning, because clinical reasoning and social life dissolve into one another, remaking therapeutics. Personal formations of healing are at odds with therapeutic practices as determined by the clinic (and indeed the clinical trial in which they were participating). Said (or asked) another way, What is the picture of healing shared by Cedric, Megan, and the clinician researchers they would see regularly? Despite the assumption that opiate-dependent adolescents are in a sense "futureless," in the case of Cedric and Megan we are forced to contend with personal forecasting and an almost overdetermined picture of a dependency-free future. Cedric and Megan actively work against the idea that substance abuse is a chronic, lifelong condition, but they acknowledge the pitfalls of recovery through a suspicion of one another. The commonly held picture of the addiction treatment career cycle (periods of relapse, treatment reentry, recovery, incarceration, abstinence in the community, and possibly death) did not hold for them.[34] Instead, they held onto something singular: a future directed by their commitment to the therapy.

WAYNE

The relationship that Wayne had with Cedric and Megan is hard to characterize as one clear type. He procured drugs for them, but strictly speaking he was not their drug dealer. He was a friend, but remained aloof and seemed to take pleasure in straining the relationship between the two of them. He would drive a wedge between Cedric and Megan at one moment, and be the person that held them together in the next. I overheard more than one conversation by phone where it was clear that Wayne was on the other end convincing either Megan or Cedric that one was in love with the other. When he came into their lives, Megan had only just begun using pills and heroin. Wayne was part of an initiation into drug use, and Cedric passively went along with Wayne's direction.

Speaking with Wayne was difficult. He rarely made eye contact, and when he did engage it was almost always to challenge or to manipulate. He would insist that I give him money (I refused repeatedly), or, when I offered Megan and Cedric rides to the clinic or other places, he would either try to tag along or ask to be taken to some distant destination ("Drive me to [Washington] DC, okay? Just tell 'em it's for your work.").

While the tension that Wayne caused between Cedric and Megan was very real, there was also something profoundly intimate about their mutual relationships. Wayne could be calming to both Cedric and Megan when they were around him. Each shared the suspicion that the other was having sex with Wayne. It was never entirely voiced as such, but there was a history within the relationship that I could never access and that was somehow out of bounds for discussion.

The role that Wayne played in "schooling" Cedric and Megan about drug use was bound up with the precision of their self-medication, *self-therapeutics*. He offered advice to both of them throughout. He also seemed to have knowledge of the treatment center and how replacement therapy worked, but perhaps more importantly, what should be "said and not said" when Cedric would return for refills of his prescription of buprenorphine and counseling. Concealment and the management of what others are able to see were strategies Wayne used both socially and institutionally. Wayne helped Cedric and Megan manage the frequency of dosage, and other details that cannot be taken for granted even in the clinical context.[35] Not knowing the long-term outcomes of the treatment included the lack of any clear understanding of the best dosage and tapering of the drug over time.[36] In many ways, Cedric and Megan were managing the uncertainty of the treatment in a fashion similar to the clinic (test, observe, change) though there were many more substances and circumstances in play.

In the one conversation I had with Wayne, when I drove him to a repair shop to pick up his frequently broken-down car, I asked for his thoughts on Cedric and Megan's program of recovery:

> You know, they trying something, so that's better than most of these fuckers out here. Junkies be junkies. If they [Cedric and Megan] junkies, they'd be junkies already. You born with the gene, you know? Someday they'll walk into that fucking rehab and say, "Hey, I'm clean, so fuck you!"

I also asked Wayne what he thought about the "chart" Cedric and Megan kept. He laughed: "Don't believe everything you read."

READING THE PAPER

The media accounts regarding the abuse and diversion of buprenorphine became a technology of suspicion, and a hugely effective one at that. When I discussed the articles with many of the actors who either wrote or publicly commented on them, their stories remained almost entirely the same. I expected more nuance, more ambiguity, and in some way a less polemical stance on all sides. As a well-known addiction medicine specialist in Philadelphia told me (an expert the reporters sought as a source), "the reporters were on a crusade" and little could deter them from the kind of story they wanted to tell. Not only was this the case, but the local media accounts in Baltimore also moved outward into national media outlets, reestablishing and amplifying the story again and again.

I carried the articles around for weeks after they were published, hoping to share them with the clinicians and residential staff at the treatment center. I even mentioned the articles in my telephone survey with healthcare providers certified by SAMHSA to prescribe buprenorphine on an outpatient basis. At the residential treatment center, the articles represented a threat—a threat to the standard of care that had been created with the new therapy, and an indictment of the program itself. A psychiatrist at the treatment center, who would later become a friend and collaborator, was very direct in her response: "They [the reporters] have no idea what they're talking about. It's good fiction, but bad fact," simultaneously signaling their absurdity while recognizing the impact the articles seemed to have. As simple as it was, her response was the most reasonable I had heard. She had little patience to respond to the details of diversion and abuse that the articles claimed. "We've got bigger problems to deal with, namely, how to keep kids on the medication and off street drugs." I asked if she ever suspected that any of the adolescents she treated were either selling or abusing buprenorphine. "No, I don't ask. I really don't need to . . . you can tell if they're staying away from other opiates, or staying on the meds. . . . I always have the urinalysis."

Multiple forms of suspicion circulate around buprenorphine, put into operation by different technologies. The urinalysis is one. The chart that Cedric and Megan kept was a technology of suspicion, however faulty, about drug use outside of the arrangement they had made for themselves. The chart found in the clinic offered another technology, although the fidelity in this case is wedded to clinical medicine and lacks the intimate features of Cedric and Megan's relationship to one another, and to Wayne. It's not completely unheard of for patients to keep a diary. Often in studies, patient diaries are used to gain information about aspects of a treatment not necessarily discussed in the clinic.[37] The "chart" that Cedric and Megan kept was different, however. It was not to be shared; it was meant to record something that was delicate in their relationship: a shared conception of therapeutics.

A short time after they were published, I brought the articles from *The Baltimore Sun* over to Cedric's house, to hear his thoughts and perhaps to complain a little about the contents. Cedric quietly read the articles with some interest at first, and then handed the small stack of papers back to me: "Figures that some fiends be doing that. Drug addicts are stupid and criminal." After handing the stack of papers back to me, Cedric asked if I wanted to come with him to his next outpatient therapy session and whether I'd take him to refill his prescription. Knowing that he planned to continue "diverting and misusing" the medication, I couldn't help but comment on the dissonance. "Isn't what you're doing kind of similar to what the paper is complaining about?" Without hesitation, he responded "No." Staying on the prescription of Suboxone—in whatever form—paradoxically gave Cedric and Megan the sense that their drug use remained faithfully under the sign of therapeutics. Between public and private dilemmas, between the extremely porous categories of *licit* and *illicit* drug use that the newspaper articles seemed to miss, there was nothing ambiguous about therapy for Cedric and Megan.

5 / PATIENTHOOD

P ATIENTHOOD IS ASSIGNED AND TAKEN UP IN DIFFERENT FORMS OUT-
side the clinical environment. Patienthood is carried into different
domains by patients—and that alone requires some elaboration (specula-
tion) on how patienthood is formed. My aim, however, is not to trace out
the many ways adolescents *performed* patienthood outside the treatment
center in the various settings where they found themselves. Certainly, Ty
had a complicated way of negotiating his HIV status, his addiction, and his
sense of personhood inside and outside environments where his conditions
were well known. Jeff held to a very definite idea of who (what) the adolescent patient-addict was, something that he actively sought to avoid or get
out from under. Simply to note all the times adolescents *talked* like patients
when they were not directly under treatment strikes me as already overdetermined. Instead, I'd like to suggest that the way the adolescents I followed
would maintain (and sometimes cultivate) themselves as objects of medical
intervention is tied up with a projection, although sometimes a seriously
disjointed one, shared between themselves and the medical practitioners
they encountered.

A PHILOSOPHY IN AND OF MEDICINE

Medical work at the residential treatment center does not need to begin with
a philosophy *of* medicine in order to perform its functions. I realize such a
statement may, at the very least, chafe the sensibilities of anthropologists,
historians, and physicians alike. Let me explain. I say this because there is
already a philosophy *in* medicine as it is performed in the clinic, *in* its practices, a philosophy that guides practitioners as well as patients through a
process of therapy and recovery.[1] Whether or not such a philosophy is articulated as such is beside the point—for better or worse, a philosophy *of* medi-

cine is there *in the doing* of medical work. As one physician at the residential treatment center continually reminded me, "Doctors here *put out* fires. We don't just *think* about fires."

Byron Good has shown in great detail how medical education serves to teach physicians to conceptualize patients as objects upon which work is performed, through the mastering of various styles of speaking, touching, and writing.[2] Patients are problems to be solved. Good's observations regarding the stakes of pedagogy in medicine and the professionalization of clinical sensibilities are important, yet in the specific case of addiction therapy I have a growing uneasiness with the distance placed between the medical practitioner and the patient. There seems to be a shadowy place where the transactions of reasoning between doctor and patient have been obscured. Cedric and Megan certainly reside in this shadow. The individual patient can (and often does) take up medical tropes. For instance, doctors and patients share a mutual reliance on terms borrowed from evidence-based medicine to make *individual, subjective* health and disorder meaningful, even in the most pedestrian way. As others have observed, in contemporary evidence-based medicine the concept of health adheres to standard values for populations.[3] At the other extreme—and as liberating as theories of individual health can be (I am thinking here of Nietzsche's *The Gay Science*)—the transactions of the body in sickness, located in language and action, are also about negotiating *concepts* across the apparent chasm separating the individual and the collective.

Mark Letteri, in an essay on the theme of health in Nietzsche's thought, writes that there is no "will to health alone."[4] Nietzsche underscores again and again that sickness is the evidence of a struggle that is the essence of health. The value of this struggle (as with life itself) cannot be estimated, because it is unknown as much as "others" are unknown, and because this value arises from the individual.[5] The notion of health in Nietzsche arises from an individual's struggle over the vast confusion of contradictory drives. Letteri writes, "The idea of power without the notion of friction is empty; consequently, [quoting Nietzsche] *'the will to power* [to health] can manifest itself only against resistances; therefore it seeks that which resists it.' "[6] Resistance is a *(the)* capacity (the *fitness*) of the individual, in overcoming sickness, to learn from it.

If resistance is the starting point for understanding the movements of sickness and health, where does this leave the *patient*? The patient is neither solely a subject-position occupied by the person experiencing illness or disorder, nor purely an object of medical intervention; rather, *the patient is a category of thought*. I have tried weighing this argument carefully against my anthropological engagements, namely, in how the patient as a producer of knowledge of disorder (as a research subject) is simultaneously an object of that knowledge when physicians perform their clinical work. Stated differently, it is difficult to locate the precise moment when and where a patient is both object and subject of research science and clinical practice, and when and where this double position can no longer be abstracted away from the lived realities of the experience of treatment for various actors.

In the clinic, the roles of the researcher (to monitor research subjects) and that of the clinician (to treat patients) are not completely separate. Something I encountered again and again was the ability on the part of the physicians to manage their dual roles, as well as to straddle the competing sets of values, methods, and expectations that come with being both deeply invested clinicians and dispassionate researchers. From a distance, there seems to be a serious discrepancy between the *clinical* lens and the *research* lens, yet in the end, as one physician shared with me, "It doesn't change the standard of care and how we see [here, meaning to treat] patients." In the residential treatment center, the "patient" (as a subject of knowledge in research and an object of intervention in medical care) is an ambiguous category, determined by the way diagnoses are *made* and medical care is *offered*. In part, the ambiguity derives from a basic conflict between the individual experience of therapeutics and the accumulation of discrete forms of evidence (facts) put in service of understanding and addressing disorder more generally. To put it more plainly, there is a conflict between individual, subjective health on the one hand, and collective, public health (and with it, evidence-based medicine) on the other.[7]

As discussed earlier, when the nurse practitioner associated with a research study in the clinic spoke to me about paying attention to the things that surround clinical practice and therapeutic offering, the nondiscursive indications of a therapy's effectiveness (affect, comportment, mannerism, drooling, maybe acting out and throwing a chair at a staff member) then become discursive—they are discussed at length every day in the staff room at the clinic. "Our research questions miss *so* much. We only hope that everything lines up in the end," she told me. The fact that *things* surrounding clinical practice cannot find a place along the continuum of research conducted in the same environment (and with the same *subjects*) is telling. Clinician researchers can only "hope" that the results of the research study align with the realities of treatment and care. But even more revealing is how these "things" fail to find a proper grammar in the research narrative, turning the realities of day-to-day medical care into abstractions. In this context, the "clinical" (as the event of treatment) is held apart from the aims of research science. Such distances represent the parsimony research science requires, and the clinic denies.

THE PATIENT AS A CATEGORY OF THOUGHT

There is something in the shadow of the experience of therapy that remakes the meaning of therapeutics. Looking at the blending of worlds outside the clinic with the values and practices within is different from assigning a random end point and then reading backward through a set of clinical criteria to judge either the success or failure of a given therapy. There is, however, an important question that remains unanswered: What does it mean to represent patienthood? Here I am not attempting to suggest some general theory of what (or who) a patient *is* or *is not*—such an exercise would be completely empty. Instead, I want to examine how the category of the patient is inhabited and lived, especially at a time, at least in America, where "being a patient" does not always guarantee medical intervention, and where diagnostics not only direct treatment, but also make treatment possible. How is it that through the category of the patient the meanings of sickness and health, even on an economic and political level, are constantly reshaped? When young men and women find themselves in residential drug treatment, it is not difficult to take on the role of the addict-as-patient. "It comes with the territory," one clinician told me. Over and over, I witnessed how the category of the adolescent drug addict was inhabited (by the adolescents themselves) and remade (by adolescents, by parents, by clinicians, and by media). At first glace, the role of the addict was something *acted* and *performed* by adolescents in the residential treatment center as *mise-en-scène*. It was only through protracted interactions with these adolescents that the role (and the idea of "performance") slowly gave way to something unpredictable, something more complicated and ultimately more telling of the experience of drug-dependence treatment, and with it the experience of patienthood. However the designation of the addict-as-patient was clung to tightly in group therapy, in individual treatment, and in the informal interactions between clinical staff and residents. It was also embedded in the routines of treatment center itself.[8]

"The addict" was not a stand-alone category of patienthood at the treatment center. There were other designations of patienthood that would compete for ascendancy: the assignment of psychiatric diagnoses would often be at odds with the diagnosis of drug dependency and vice versa. Drawing a distinction between "being crazy" and "being a dope fiend" was a strategy used by doctors and nurses to secure funding for an adolescent's stay at the treatment center. The adolescents would also adopt these designations (something administrative as much as clinical) to define their "disorders" throughout time in treatment.[9] Over the many hours of conversation I had with one of the intake nurses, a middle-aged man who had worked for several years in the "burnout" position of intake coordinator, he was frank about what diagnoses meant:

> It is never far from the truth, throwing a DSM-IV [*Diagnostic and Statistical Manual of Mental Disorders-DSM IV*] number down on paper. But to Blue Cross/Blue Shield [a common private health insurance utilized in treatment], or other health insurers, it is serious business. It's a game of guessing what they're looking for and playing along. In the end, all the kids get the treatment they need, more or less. There's not one kid in here that isn't suffering from both [having psychiatric and dependency comorbidities].

The order of the diagnoses was immensely important. Was a psychologically disturbed adolescent *self-medicating* with illicit substances to manage her disorder? Should she be "routed" to a psychiatric hospital rather than admitted into residential drug-dependency treatment? If so, was there a chance she would be denied treatment at the psychiatric hospital, as well? The language used by the nurses was also hugely important when describing how a patient "presented." And yet, regardless of the severity—regardless of the diagnosis—the argument for "medical necessity" was often not enough to overcome the limitations of public and private health insurance, and adolescents were turned away.

Diagnoses were not benign—nor were they random or hidden. They were known, interpreted, and used in various ways by parents, staff, and the other adolescents under treatment. Newly admitted adolescents would sit in a chair in the small intake room on the first floor, sometimes for hours, even while feeling the effects of withdrawal, waiting for their stay at the treatment center to be bartered over the telephone with private insurers or with public aid administrators. The intake room was where I first met Jeff, dissolving into a sweaty pool of opiate withdrawal before my eyes. He attempted to sit stoically in a chair and wait. Hours later, between intermittent periods of nodding off and shaking, Jeff was finally admitted into detoxification. What was obvious *in the flesh* was meticulously relayed in words by the nurse to the person with the power to authorize an admission on the other end of the telephone. It is important to emphasize that the diagnostic strategies used by the nurses were not about fictionalizing disorder to create treatment opportunities, but rather that the process of naming (and, in a sense, concealing) disorder exposes the porous boundaries between elements of discrete symptomatology (how things are felt and seen) and their signification (how things are described and valued).[10]

The definition of a patient may at first seem stable: one who suffers from some ailment, either known or unknown—one who becomes ill and seeks a return to a former state.[11] But the given-ness of such a definition (the return to a former state) is up for grabs when considered against the lived realities of care, healing, and self-knowledge. The patient is a subject that resides between the individual and the social under the corresponding signs of sickness and health. Moreover, the patient figures as the normative ground between sickness and health; the patient is the ground upon which healing and intervention stake their meaning. But if the patient—at once a workable object and the subject of disease—is a ground, it is *terra incognita*. In his description of disease as understood through the clinic's reorientation to the body, Foucault writes:

> From the point of view of death, disease has a land, a mappable
> territory, a subterranean but secure place where its kinships and its
> consequences are formed; local values define its forms. Paradoxically,
> the presence of the corpse enables us to perceive it living—living
> with a life that is no longer that of either old sympathies or the

combinative laws of complications, but one that has its own roles and its own laws.[12]

The secured and singular place where disease takes hold is a cohabitation *with* and *within* the living body. The reformulation does not undermine the force of Foucault's observation; it changes its terms. It needs to be said, however, that the ground upon which "disease" and the sick "body" are founded inside the clinic (and especially outside the clinic) is perhaps a more complicated and less *mappable* territory than Foucault suggests. What kinships chart the living body? Or what, as Arthur Frank asks, authorizes medicine to claim the living body as its territory?[13] The patient does more than provide information about her ailing body; the patient does more than act, somewhat paradoxically, as a disarticulation of her own corporeal geography. Yet the construction of the patient–disease relation has been gradually imposed and naturalized within biomedicine. In a short essay entitled "Diseases," Canguilhem writes:

> [T]he patient-disease [*malade-maladie*] relation cannot be of complete
> discordance. In contemporary societies, where medicine endeavors
> to become a science of diseases, the institutions of public health and
> the popularization of medical knowledge have the effect that, for the
> patient, living his disease means also talking and hearing talk in clichés
> or stereotypes; living his disease means implicitly valorizing the results
> of a knowledge whose progress is due in part to putting the patient
> between brackets, however much he may be the avowed subject of
> medical concern.[14]

The process of bracketing the patient is not about descriptive precision, nor is it an attempt to ascribe the necessary characteristics to the patient as a subject per se; instead, it is a particular way of inserting a distinction between the normal and the pathological.[15] This much is clear. But it is also a matter of putting words—"talking and hearing talk"—to experience. Putting words to experience, to illness, to pain, to exact its prose is precisely the thing that allows the language of the patient–disease relation to run dry.[16] Even in accounts where the word and the body are so closely (yet so distantly) aligned—where experience and expression are produced from within—there is the specter of a failure when attempting to "represent" illness.[17]

Stated very simply, the medical encounter is always (at the very least) a two-way encounter, two medical events, which together produce and shape meaning.[18] Yet bodily experience and medical imagination are not simply disparate points of view.[19] What appear to be vantage points are places that mark opposing concepts, making visible (audible) the way such concepts are enunciated and thereby resonate into one another. Canguilhem observed that ordinary concepts are utterly unavailable to the sick man, that it is "impossible for the physician, starting from the accounts of sick men, to understand the experience lived by the sick man, for what sick men express in ordinary concepts is not directly their experience but their interpretation of an experience for which they have been deprived of adequate concepts."[20] Inadequate concepts are the very foundation for expressing the bodily experience of sickness.

Within a clinical framework, uncertainty is replaced by diagnostic and conceptual precision—and yet uncertainty is the very thing transmitted across the thin threshold between *health* and *illness*, the very thing transmitted between medicine and its object. Where, then, is the ground on which this transmission between medicine and the body takes place? Where is the place from which illness is unmoored from the living body? The concern I raise is what it means to live with (and through) illness and how life comes to be mediated by medical intervention. To borrow some phrasing from Veena Das, the experience of illness condenses and collapses a network of meaning, giving expression to a particular pattern of life that sickness threatens to dissolve.[21] However, although Das describes this "condensing and collapsing" of meaning, the problem in the case of adolescents in drug-dependency treatment is how to give expression to the pattern of life remade through illness in ethnographic telling, beyond the terms offered by the clinic, which nevertheless acknowledges the long reach that the clinic has. Here, the attempt (and I mean *attempt* in the strictest sense, as it is less a claim than a challenge) is to illustrate the registers through which diagnoses and medical work produce and give meaning to individual and social realities beyond what is considered strictly neutral medical knowledge.[22]

SOME ROUGH ACCOUNTING

There is no way to account for all the turns in treatment, both inside and outside the clinic. The focus on an individual is not simply a methodological strategy or ethnographic convention. One case is not meant to move seamlessly into the next. The attention to the individual exposes the multiplicity that already exists within diagnostic categories. Merleau-Ponty identified this understanding of the individual in the work of Kurt Goldstein: "Instead of considering the same symptom in many subjects, he addresses himself to the complete analysis of one single subject, striving to explore all areas of behavior."[23] I maintain that to look into the lives of young men and women through the *place* of patienthood—where diagnoses are offered and taken up—*cuts to the core* of the individual experience of patienthood. The space of the clinic, its *milieu*, joins with what is *clinical* (as an analytical perspective), together working to shape the *experience* of a diagnostic category. Along similar lines, it is difficult to ignore Gilbert Simondon's *L'individu et sa genèse physico-biologique* (The Individual and His Physico-Biological Genesis), wherein he makes clear the distinction between individuality and singularity. In the work of Simondon, the individual is not necessarily a given, but is in a sense *naturalized* (in the specific cases I describe, *naturalized* as a medical subject through diagnostics and therapeutic intervention).[24]

The patient is not strictly an object of medical knowledge, nor the subject of disorder, but a category of thought that is negotiated within medicine and therapeutics, inside and outside the clinic. Here, claims to the efficacy and effectiveness of a therapy—and to the process of therapeutics more generally—must attend, in the strictest sense, to *what is seen, what is spoken or attested to, and what is lived*.

6 / DISAPPEARANCES

THE DISAPPEARANCE OF SUBJECTS IN AN ETHNOGRAPHY OF ADDIC-tion does not offer closure or finality to the ethnographic encounter but instead raises difficult questions regarding the stakes and values inherent in anthropological work—perhaps especially work that takes as its object disorder and suffering. Two of the adolescents I followed died and two others became lost to me in the tangle of clinical and criminal-legal institutions in Baltimore. Rather than taking death and loss as tropes to frame and organize meaning in the lives of these adolescents, I suggest that addiction and treatment—and their aftermath—force a broader definition of self-care as a technology of living, one that recognizes that the conditions of *a life* must incorporate the lived realities of local moral worlds and, at times, severely constrained agency at the level of the individual.

DISAPPEARANCES

I want to address the *problems* and *realities* of disappearance in an ethnography of addiction. In the clinic and other environments through which I would follow adolescents receiving treatment for drug dependency, my interactions were episodic and often unpredictable. It was not uncommon for there to be one or two months between the times I would connect with the young men and women I was attempting to follow. For my part, the times in between were filled with anxiety and the promise of failure. There was no guarantee that I would see or talk with them again. Every interaction, whether a conversation in a living room or a shared meal in the treatment center cafeteria, felt like it might be the last.

Disappearance is a *problem* in an ethnography of adolescents abusing drugs not because it shatters the illusion of continuity in the ethnographic encounter, but because it foregrounds a set of concerns regarding the values and assumptions shared between anthropological and clinical work, complicating what would otherwise be a straightforward narrative of addiction, recovery, and very often relapse. Disappearance is a *reality* because it reflects the conditions and circumstances in the lives of individuals that require centering on the pages of anthropological writing. I'm thinking especially of Arthur Kleinman's formulation of "writings at the margin," which not only signals overlapping disciplinary commitments, but also helps to locate something near the edge of experience that nevertheless becomes central to anthropological writing itself.[1]

LIFE AND THOUGHT

The headings "technologies of the self" and "the care of the self" have given anthropology—for a long time now—the space to move out from under previous frameworks of selfhood or personhood. Anthropologists have challenged psychologically centered ideas of selfhood by showing how moral and historical exteriority is folded inward at the level of the individual,[2] and by calling for more nuanced renderings of subjectivity, although these are nevertheless "riddled by structural forces, cultural sensibilities, subjective vicissitudes, political tensions, pragmatic forces, and rhetorical pitches."[3] The individual experience of therapy can be articulated, in the terms Michel Foucault offers, as the formation of subjectivity by the individual as the condition of self-care.[4] However, the nature of the individual (subject, person, self)—as an object of study—needs to be clear. The distinction between "the individual" as a general category and "the individuated subject" as (someone) singular is best articulated in the works of Gilles Deleuze and Gilbert Simondon. To talk about the experience of therapeutics as "self-care" is to speak of the individuated subject.[5] However, just as the (medical) subject comes under different headings, *life* comes under different headings as well. What does it mean to be human, or, more specifically, to make claims *of* the living? To talk about the value and worth of *life* is to speak about the value of *a life*.[6]

To follow the argument from the introduction of Georges Canguilhem's *Knowledge of Life*, *thought* and the *living* are not separate or contradictory, but come to rest upon one another—nothing of life absents itself or is unmade by thought.[7] Yet, as both François Dagognet[8] and Georges Canguilhem[9] have shown, there is an implicit split between thought and living (knowledge and life) in research science and clinical medicine. Life is an object examined from the outside. But if we turn our attention to the "speaking subject" (even when that subject is formed through techniques of confession and concealment, as Foucault argues), we find an alternative way of being that is taken up by adolescents under pharmacotherapy. *Life* and *thought* would include transformation over time, and the *experience* of therapy would do more than simply run alongside the *idea* of therapeutics.

The knowledge derived from examining treatment is not distinct from its lived experience (a difference that does not necessarily get resolved through the language of embodiment). In this way, the separation between philosophies of *experience*, of the *subject*, and of philosophies of *concepts*, *knowledge*, and *rationality* may be less distinct than Foucault suggests in his famous essay on the work of Georges Canguilhem, "Life: Experience and Science."[10] So-called authentic experience (living) is not measured against rationality (the thought of living). The transformation of thought *about* life does not unmake the experience of living. Instead it challenges the assumption of experience, in this case, the experience upon which addiction and therapeutics are predicated.[11] If therapeutic success can only be assessed on an individual level, then the value of life becomes synonymous with the values *attributed* to individual health.[12]

I am not suggesting that self-care, or more specifically the way that adolescents manage themselves in a therapeutic process, forms some kind of model of addiction experience. The creation of value (of recovery, of dwelling with drug dependency, of "making it" and "not making it") is an individual value that has the capacity to run counter to the way therapeutic interventions are imagined. Nevertheless, the clinical value of being (and remaining) under treatment becomes quickly conflated with the personal values attached to a therapy by adolescents under treatment (as well as by their families). In some ways, this is an easy observation to make. The difficulty is to avoid clumsy misattributions of *agency* in the narrative of dependency and treatment. Perhaps it is especially difficult when the illness narrative becomes the source of all knowing. Through the convention of anthropological writing, the speaking subject tells a story, one that calls attention to uncomfortable details and raises puzzling questions about *truth*, *believability*, and the *meaning of what is said*—all the while knowing that confession and concealment are not only processes of intersubjectivity, but are also the foundations of self-care.[13] The desire for continuity in ethnographic telling is not so much about *making meaning* as it is about *making sense* of things.

INTO THE INSTITUTIONAL FOLD

I came to know Keisha through her many stays in the residential treatment center. She was someone who demonstrated an inordinately difficult time negotiating home life and institutional life. I was introduced to Keisha and her mother by the outpatient coordinator, a small man with his nervous energy always directed toward his next cigarette break. He knew Keisha's mother because she had been treated for drug dependency at the center fifteen years earlier, when she was sixteen. He told me after my initial meeting with Keisha, "It makes me feel like a tree. You know? You could saw me in half and count the rings. And you'd see each generation of these girls who come in here. Mom, daughter . . . Who knows, maybe I'll meet Keisha's daughter in here some day [laughing]. Who fucking knows?"

The reunion between Keisha's mother and the outpatient coordinator was surprisingly joyful, though both her mother and the coordinator were made to suffer Keisha's irritated glare. In the months of conversations that would follow, Keisha described the interlacing roles between herself and her mother (mother, daughter, caretaker, friend, sexual competitor, disciplinarian) that were more complicated than simply one generation after the next inheriting drug dependency.[14] Keisha told me that she saw herself as "a mother to my own mother," and, at times, she took care of her younger siblings and managed the household entirely. "My moms use [drugs]. I ain't gonna lie. She be using right there in the house. And I'm like, 'Get outta here or I put your ass out.' And she'd leave with her boyfriend or whatever for, like, days. So what you gonna do? You take care of shit."

There are very distinct forms of domesticity and relatedness established around drug use, yet it is clear that this is very different from the idea that drug use forms intimacy within a network of kin.[15] Drug use was something that stressed Keisha's familial relationships and threatened the relationships that sustained the very notion of "home." Keisha and her mother seemed to fight for some kind of equilibrium relating to substance abuse, competing for care and resenting moments when care was forced upon them as the mode in which they had to relate to one another. When Keisha would abuse drugs, her mother would become furious ("crazy, a crazy hypocrite," Keisha told me). Keisha's mother kicked her out of the house several times for her drug use and was quick "to commit" Keisha to the residential treatment center during these episodes. When I asked Keisha about her mother the first time we had the chance to speak alone, she told me she was glad to be back in treatment:

> At least she can't use while I'm in here. Who take care of her kids if I ain't there? My mom gotta be a mom when I'm here. So, yeah, I'm glad. She use as soon as I'm out, which is like a slap in my face. I'm happy to be sitting right here.

Drug use was an activity that constantly reordered relationships of care and definitions of the caring between Keisha and her mother (who was being cared for and how that care was performed at a particular time). Keisha was someone who would allow herself to become folded into the system of treatment and incarceration precisely because she felt it was a way to manage the conditions of home life between stays. Keisha described her transition back into drug use precipitating her readmission to the treatment center like this:

> I'm young. I got my own life. I feel like she [her mother] trying to live my life and make my live hers. I don't want to look after her damn kids. And I don't want to be her damn mother. But shit just be that way with her. So sometimes I'm like, 'Fuck it. I wanna get high, so I get high,' and then it puts the brakes on her shit.

After several treatment episodes inside the residential treatment center, Keisha transitioned to the outpatient treatment program, where she saw a clinician once every week. I asked Keisha about the move:

> I can't take medication at home. Shit just return to normal, like before I go into rehab. My moms gonna be my moms. I get fucking tired, you know? I tell them [the clinic staff] that this ain't gonna work. But I know they ain't gonna let me hide in here forever.

Keisha returned only once to the residential treatment center after a failed attempt at outpatient treatment. She was discharged into outpatient treatment once again, though she never turned up at any of her outpatient appointments. When I contacted her mother I learned that Keisha had beaten a girl in her neighborhood so severely that the girl required hospitalization, which resulted in Keisha's arrest and incarceration. Unlike so many of the young men and women I would see pass through the residential treatment center, often lost to the neighborhoods they had come from, Keisha disappeared institutionally inward. In a certain way, she had exhausted drug rehabilitation as a way to escape her home and had dissolved into another institutional environment.

IN BETWEEN—NOWHERE

There were many disappearances out of "the system" (a term use widely by clinicians and social workers at the treatment center to capture the vastness of institutional encounters faced by the adolescents under treatment). Kevin was someone I met early on in my time at the treatment center. From the beginning my experience with him opened questions about disappearance.

When I could no longer find Kevin, he had just entered the thin divide between another set of institutions, this time the residential treatment center and home. In the past, Kevin had slipped between schools, jails, vocational training, hospitals, drug-treatment centers, foster homes, and an assortment of couches. The geography of these movements had remained relatively contained, since each move occurred in Baltimore.

When I first met Kevin it was soon after he was court-ordered to spend time at the residential drug-treatment center until his trial date (not his first, and the sense I drew from my interviews with him, possibly not his last). He had stolen his mother's truck. She pressed charges. (This, too, was not a first.) Despite turning eighteen years old in the time between the arrest and his first appearance in court, Kevin was still considered a minor. At the pretrial hearing, the judge asked Kevin if he was drunk when he stole the truck: Yes, very. The judge asked him if he was using any other substance during the incident: Yes, marijuana. There is surely more to the story. However, based on these two factors, the judge chose to put him in drug treatment rather than general holding in the juvenile criminal facility until his trial date.

During my first conversation with Kevin he described himself, sarcastically, as "a portrait of recidivism." He spoke these words with mocking perfection, yet the import they held remained out of reach; he did not quite inhabit his own speech, and instead somehow remained always on the verge (a common refrain during our conversations was that he "couldn't find the right words"). The question remains: Was Kevin "a portrait of recidivism"? No doubt. But returning again and again to what? He seemed to move organically between institutions, making him something of an institutional being, never out from under some sort of institutional gaze, ever visible through the lens of the institutions through which he passed.

On the day of Kevin's trial, his mother dropped all the charges. He was discharged from the drug-treatment facility a day later. I continued to speak with Kevin by phone and made three visits to his house in the Brooklyn neighborhood in the southernmost section of Baltimore. After a few weeks without contact, I drove over unannounced to see if I could find him at his home. The house had been demolished. When I knocked on the neighboring doors the responses I received were either vague or hostile. I called Kevin's cell phone, his mother's cell phone, and his mother's work number. Nothing, and in the last case, she had simply moved on. I contacted the Department of Corrections parole officer in charge of Kevin's case but he too had lost contact, and now that the charges had been dropped there was no way of tracking Kevin within the court system. Kevin was nowhere.

Since the age of eleven, Kevin has been arrested twenty-six times. At thirteen, he started using marijuana and hash, followed by alcohol at sixteen. When he was staying with his mother he often found himself in trouble since a lot of family members and acquaintances either just hang around the house or stay for a few weeks at a time, always seeming to get him "caught up in nonsense." The times that Kevin was arrested or institutionalized were double-edged: "Sometimes you need a vacation." I asked Kevin what it was like for him to always be tied to some institution:

> I mean, it sort of like you protected or whatever. My mom's boyfriends
> be fucking me up, beating on me . . . being assholes, taking my shit. . . .
> Like when my PO [parole officer] come around, nobody messes with me
> cause they know they be checking for shit like that. It like a one-man
> neighborhood watch or some shit.

When I asked Kevin if he had ever *not* been in some form of criminal or medical environment since his first arrest, my question was met with a blank look. Of course not—what would that even mean for Kevin, given the frequency and breadth of his institutional life, one seemingly without start or finish? "It's all the same," he told me. The last interview we had together, I made a joke, saying that he makes my job too easy in that I can always find him. He laughed and said, "My life is an open book. I'm like the Yellow Pages."

Through Kevin's story I take up two questions, one clinical and one ethnographic. First, what does it mean to be a part of a therapeutic process (and here I'm referring specifically to drug-dependency treatment) that happens so rapidly, that is, one marked by constant change as well as the changing loci of the thing being "treated"? And second, what are the limits of "visibility" *within* and *between* institutions? Somewhere lingering between these two questions is also a concern about the reliance on certain institutions to provide the necessary "access" to individuals for ethnographic work to be made possible.

One version of Kevin's story was his case history, held neatly in the pages of his treatment chart. According to his chart, Kevin had been diagnosed with ADHD (Attention Deficit Hyperactivity Disorder) and bipolar disorder. Throughout his past nine in-patient hospitalizations and one outpatient treatment, he had been prescribed Seroquel (a drug indicated for the treatment of schizophrenia as well as for the treatment of acute manic episodes associated with bipolar disorder, taken as an adjunct therapy to lithium). Kevin had had several psychiatric hospitalizations, which he describes as "total meltdowns." "Sometimes things just be too stressful, you know, and something gotta give." In one case, he was in line at a Chinese carryout in his mother's neighborhood. In line he began punching the air wildly, "like I was fighting some army," and somehow, though he claims he wanted to, he couldn't stop. Finally the police arrived, calmed him, and took him directly to an emergency room: "They just like dropped me off at they doorstep, and told 'em 'he's nuts.' They gave me a shot and that really fucked me up . . . I really felt nuts." He had seen several psychiatrists during these periods of hospitalization, but never remembered the names of his physicians or the situations in which any pharmaceuticals continued to be prescribed. When I asked him whether or not he felt he was suffering from some form of mental illness, he answered with a question: "Do you even know how these places round here break down the mind?" From our first meeting at the drug treatment center, a persistent topic driving conversations was that different factors were constantly at play in either keeping him "straight" or "fucking with" him. Kevin never really discussed his drug use, which by all accounts was fairly mild compared to many of his fellow residents at the treatment center. Drug use and abuse seemed to be a switch that Kevin used to manage other situations (internal and external).

There were other clinical concerns as well. During his last episode of treatment, Kevin tested positive for *Chlamydia trachomatis*. During our conversations it became clear that he had been treated for both gonorrhea and chlamydia in the past (both at the Baltimore Health Department STD Clinic). Kevin claimed to have been tested for HIV many times, but never bothered to return for his results (or did not wish to discuss this with me). "Fuck it, I'm clean." Kevin also wheezed during every conversation we had, and while I was always reluctant to ask about this, he used the insult "weak ass, asthma motherfuckers" to describe other residents at the treatment center more than once, giving some odd indication of a kind of self-awareness.

So what is the issue? A drug-treatment center, like any number of clinical environments, is a place where multiple medical concerns come to light— through the systemization of screening and diagnostics directed toward specific diseases (largely communicable) and disorders (largely psychiatric). And while such things are important to document (ethnographically and otherwise), pointing out this fact does not represent a tremendous insight. But here something entirely different is happening. Diagnoses do adhere to individuals as they pass through various medico-legal environments, yet in this case the disorder at hand, made most pressing given the institutional context, tends to establish an order for all other disorders. When Kevin is hospitalized for some incident, whether it's an outburst in a Chinese carry-out or, in another case, sitting for hours starring blankly at a shopping mall food court, he is—foremost—a psychiatric patient. When he does something that involves drugs or alcohol, he is a substance-abusing teenager. When he shows up repeatedly at the STD clinic, he is labeled high-risk for HIV. It would be a mistake to assume that these forms of designation never intersect, but understanding how they intersect—how these "reorderings" are mapped onto something called medical experience—is exceedingly important. This also invites (forces) a completely different conceptualization of comorbidity. Where one notion of comorbidity assumes that disorders occur simultaneously or in concert with one another, here disorders are marked and ordered in terms of an external rubric of importance, in serial form. In the clinic, whether or not a particular situation requires medical assistance through a third-party payer (or whether treatment is free) is also a key element of this ordering. Kevin rarely remained in any given program long enough for these designations to come together to form some cogent understanding, or to reveal something underlying that would bind the things he experiences together, clinically or otherwise.

INTO THE FOLD OF FAMILY

Two of the adolescents that I followed died. Their deaths occurred months after the last time I spoke with either of them at the clinic and the variety of environments they called home. The deaths forced me to rethink many things, not least of which was how to write about their deaths in a way that would not evacuate the content of their stories, or—more dangerously—orient their stories toward the inevitability of dying.

Tanya was from Baltimore County and her home was not far from the residential treatment center. The first thing I noticed about her was how much younger she looked compared to the other girls of her age in treatment. She was precocious and completely self-assured. Tanya spoke with a slightly southern drawl, having spent many summers with extended family in West Virginia and Delaware. In the months leading up to a drug-possession charge and admission into the treatment center, she had begun snorting and smoking heroin with her boyfriend.

Tanya loathed residential treatment and hated the confinement and routine of institutional life. She wanted to make a home for herself outside the restrictive atmosphere of the treatment center. Tanya expressed a desire for independence, yet she would describe at great length her dependence upon and complicated relationship with her boyfriend: "He's good to me, you know. He doesn't put hands on me or nothing. We get fighting sometime, but you know, who don't?" She talked at length about sex with her boyfriend and her sexual history in a way that was clearly meant to offer evidence of her boyfriend's love for her. There was something desperate in the way she gave evidence to the care in her relationship. Her eagerness was complicated by the fact that she gave every indication that there was something amiss in the relationship. She would leave some statements about her boyfriend intentionally vague: "He ain't a pimp. He'd never force me to do anything I don't wanna do. I mean, he lets me make my own choices about things. Maybe I do what he say, but it's still my choice."

Tanya broke up with her boyfriend two months after she was discharged from the residential treatment center. Almost immediately after she was discharged, they had begun using together again, and at some point he became violent and insisted that she trade sex for drugs or money to support their mutual habit. She refused and he beat her—badly. He burned her clothes in the bathtub before he left the apartment and smashed the windows of a car she had borrowed from a friend. Tanya told me the details of the incident weeks after it had happened. She held a cigarette cupped in her hand and recounted the details through the thin trail of smoke rising from between her fingers. We were sitting on the bench outside a convenience store in a light rain, around the corner from the new place she was staying:

> That bitch landlord kicked me out. The fire department had to come and put out the fire, and the next day I got put out. "I found drug paraphernalia," she told me, but I know it was the fire department coming what done it. I know she thinks I'm a whore, too. Fuck her. I hope her daughter gets what happened to me. Who puts out a girl with a beat-up face?

In a strange twist, it was her boyfriend's aunt who took Tanya in. "I had no clothes, and he stole my purse on his way out with all my money and ID and stuff in it. He left me for dead [laughing]. She [the ex-boyfriend's aunt] always liked me, like a daughter I guess." Several weeks passed before the next time we spoke. We agreed to meet again at the convenience store around the corner from the aunt's house for take-out food. Tanya was already there, sitting on a bench. I did not recognize her at first. She was much thinner, which was hard to imagine given how small she was to begin with. She was wearing an oversized sweatshirt, and her face had sunken. Her fingers were brownish yellow from nicotine. When I returned from ordering food, I was blunt: "Are you shooting up?" Tanya gave a shrug of indifference and was equally blunt with her answer: "Yeah."

Tanya was taken in by a group of older women at the aunt's house. She began injecting heroin almost immediately from the time she moved in with them. "It was like a gift, you know? A welcome home gift, like 'this is where you belong.'" I asked her how she was making money to support herself, but she wouldn't say (and I did not press the issue). She said that she was no longer allowed in the convenience store after being caught shoplifting, which explained part of her nervousness while talking with me on the bench in front of the store. She looked up and down the street as we spoke, as though she was waiting for (or trying to avoid) someone.

I had no way of contacting her after her cell phone was cut off. I went by the house a few times, but there was never an answer at the door. A few months after we last spoke, I found a contact number for her stepfather who lived in Delaware in her chart at the clinic. When I spoke with him he told me that Tanya had died from complications related to an overdose a month earlier, and he abruptly hung up the phone.

RECOVERY AND LOSS

Jeff stopped using drugs altogether. After a few weeks at the treatment center and one month of outpatient therapy, he stopped treatment altogether, too. "I'm clean. I don't take drugs, not even weed. I'm back," he told me as we drove to his house from the corner where he instructed me to pick him up. "It's like I'm a different person, you know? You got to be. I got no room for mistakes. I got money, I earned my place and it ain't easy."

Jeff was shot and killed little more than three months from the time he left the residential treatment center. It is unclear if a drug sale went badly or if he was fighting with another dealer. According to his cousin, who had been the person that helped me to stay in contact with Jeff after he left the treatment center, Jeff was shot twice in the head. "He didn't see it coming. One minute you're here, and then nothing. He didn't see himself go, I'm sure of it," Jeff's cousin told me. The funeral had happened a week before I called Jeff's cousin, hoping to talk to Jeff again despite the fact that in our last conversation it was clear that he did not want to see me again. I drove to Jeff's cousin's house and he drove me to the graveyard. There were pink silk flowers on the top of a modest granite tombstone—a tombstone that had space for three more names and dates. The tombstone had his family name and his first name carved below, with the date of his birth: 1991. It struck me how young he was when he died. Jeff's cousin asked if I could make a donation to help cover the funeral costs, which were still outstanding. "Of course." It was all I could think to say.

The last conversation I had with Jeff was brief. He had reestablished himself on the street. He was clean. He had hardened. He didn't want to continue talking with me, though I told myself that it was simply that he didn't want to be around someone who reminded him of his (in his words) "past life" as an addict. "When you clean, you clean. That's it. Nothing else to discuss." Jeff asserted himself in a way that demanded the disconnection from addiction and treatment. I was able to ask him a few questions the last time I saw him. He made little eye contact during our brief conversation:

> TODD: So, do you regret taking the medication (buprenorphine)? Do you
> think it worked?

> JEFF: Worked? Fuck that. I *worked*. You gotta work if you wanna rid
> your body and mind of that shit. Ain't no pill going *work* for you.
> People be lazy.

> TODD: Okay. So, do you think you'll ever need to go back into treat-
> ment? I mean relapse, or something? Or even just for support?

> JEFF: Why? You don't think I worked hard enough to get off the shit?
> I'll be right here, doing my thing. Fuck. *You* go back. I ain't.

In whatever way, Jeff was successful in his efforts to wean himself from opiates. Tanya fell into a pattern of drug use that eventually ended her life. In both cases there are details not easily reconciled. Tanya found a group of women who took her in during a moment of crisis. She found a home. There was a deep intimacy and care in the way she described these women, and a kinship she felt with them. Jeff's abstinence from drugs of any kind allowed him to return to his previous place selling drugs on the corner. With the return to dealing, he had to assert himself to regain his former place and status. Though his cousin never said it directly, it was implied that Jeff had shot someone to reestablish a level of credibility.

In each of these accounts—Jeff, Keisha, Kevin, and Tanya—there is something in the shadow of the experience of therapy that remakes the meaning of therapeutics, but there is even more here about the way *living* is unexpectedly folded into the narrative of addiction and recovery. It is one thing to claim that the lifeworlds outside the clinic are blended with the values and practices within the clinic. But it is perhaps more important to be reminded of the impossibility of taking the end point of addiction and the therapeutic process as the point from which to judge either the success or failure of a therapy—or whether life followed a desired course, one that can be valued positively or negatively only in retrospect. Jeff was a pharmacotherapeutic success. He was clean and intended to stay clean. Tanya was an utter failure, having deepened her drug abuse. In the end, the outcomes were the same.

OF CONTINUITY AND RUPTURE

The adolescents I followed challenged the idea of continuity in ethnographic work, or at least forced a rethinking of the concept. This is not to say that medical anthropology suffers from a lack of awareness when it comes to rupture or discontinuity, but in an ethnography of drug dependence and treatment these concerns are particularly poignant. For instance, I did not expect to lose touch with Cedric and Megan so abruptly. Megan always talked about getting out of Baltimore. Cedric thought he and Megan would leave together. I never found out. He moved out of his mother's house, and she didn't know (or was unwilling to say) where he had gone. I called and stopped by Megan's mother's house, where she would often see her younger siblings, but she had not been there to visit in several weeks. Megan's mother claimed Megan would come back, but who knows. I hoped I would see Cedric at outpatient meetings, but he neglected to show up. He no longer went to the treatment center to pick up his prescription of buprenorphine.

It is surprising that adolescents whose lives are marked by such an overwhelming institutional presence move so quickly beyond or out from under these institutions. These abrupt turns raise a difficult question: What sort of reliance on forms of institutional life is anthropology—and for that matter, medicine—willing to endure? Here, my meaning is twofold. First, there is a reliance on institutions resulting from the mere practicality of *doing* ethnographic work on medical topics; and secondly, it seems impossible to dislocate institutional life from *a life* in which illness and healing are experienced. Once they leave institutional environments and the relationships originally formed there, where do adolescents like Cedric, Megan, Kevin, and Keisha go? The accounts of their experiences in and out of drug dependency treatment begin to suggest that there is something worth understanding in the shadow of anthropological work.[16] The trajectories that Jeff, Tanya, Kevin, and Keisha each followed force the shadow of their disappearances to be equally as present as what is normally seen in the light of therapeutics in the clinic.

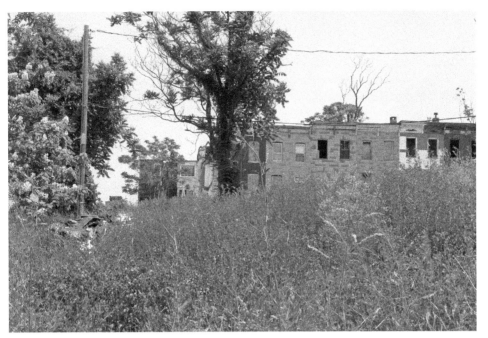

Fig. 6. Backyard of row house, southwest Baltimore.

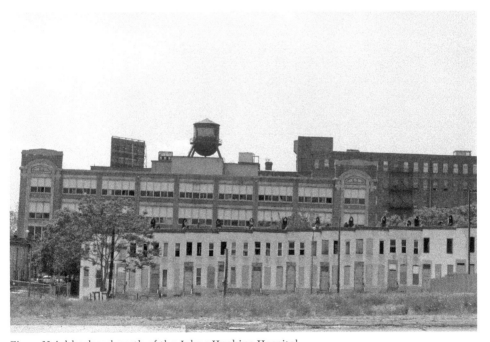

Fig. 7. Neighborhood north of the Johns Hopkins Hospital.

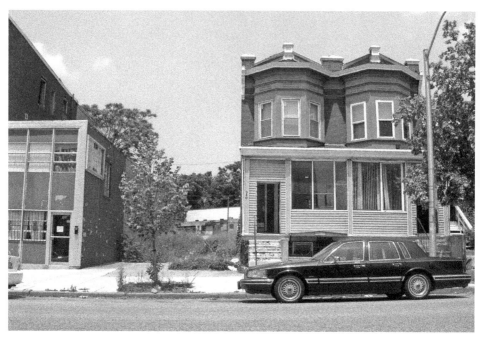

Fig. 8. East Baltimore.

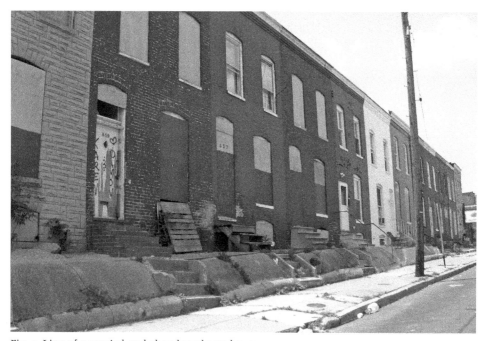

Fig. 9. Line of occupied and abandoned row houses.

CONCLUSION / ENDURING PRESENCE

I T IS DIFFICULT TO KNOW WHERE TO FIND AN ENDING. SIMPLY ASSIGN-
ing an end point at the place where adolescents disappear is not at all
satisfactory, particularly since "absence" (whether it is absence from therapy or from under the ethnographic gaze) doesn't necessarily add closure at
the end of a therapeutic episode, one generally concluded after dependency
upon opiates has been eliminated or replaced by small, sustaining doses of
therapeutic substitutes. Moreover, it seems abrupt to draw a single conclusion from the ethnography at its close. The difficulty may have to do with
a reluctance to make the claim that any one person can demonstrate either
the success or failure of treatment, a matter that speaks directly to the tension between individuated, subjective medicine and collective medicine that
forms the basis of evidence-based medicine. Making the claim of success
seems to tempt fate, begging things to career wildly off track in the future.
On the other hand, claiming failure seems to evacuate all possibility of hope.
The problem, however, is even more difficult. Again, to echo the final sen-
tence of Georges Canguilhem's essay on the pedagogy of healing, he reminds
us that hope rests perilously close to failure: "To learn to heal is to learn the
contradiction between today's hope and the defeat that comes at the end—
without saying no to today's hope."[1]

Throughout my time in the clinic, in homes, in fast-food restaurants,
sitting in waiting rooms, in kitchens, in restaurant booths, on couches, and
on front stoops, there was one question I would ask during nearly every
conversation: "How do you imagine your future?" Those who were particularly astute became progressively annoyed with the repetition and I would
reformulate the question to remain (often unsuccessfully) one step ahead
of aggravation. But in whatever form, the question was never really meant
to be about the future as such. I was much more interested in the imaginings shared by the adolescents, family members, and clinicians on what a

forecasted future might say about the present moment. I wanted to know what a picture of addiction and therapy looked like to the adolescents I spoke with—and if that picture, on whatever ground these seemingly contradictory elements occupied, could incorporate hope-laden failure, as Canguilhem suggests. In nearly every case, the answer to my question would change between conversations over many months. At times I was offered detailed imaginings of family, of children, of finding intimacy, of finding money, of living elsewhere or on one's own. At other times the imagination of a future would center much more closely on abstinence from drugs and alcohol, or more generally on being in a situation that in no way resembled the one in which they were in presently. There were also times when the answer to my question was met with a refusal to imagine any future, a response that would remain firm. From here, the future was, strictly speaking, futureless.

In conversations with the adolescents I followed, the idea of the future was about the conditions of the present. *Presence* was not cut off from the past. In fact, the past would often be called upon to help deal with the present, to explain or refute what was happening in a given moment, often pointing to some future yet to be realized. The idea of presence (as a time signature as much as just "being there") made a future possible—and with this possibility, the promise that *the future* would be a release from the present. Presence was endured and enduring.

Samuel Beckett, reflecting on the novels of Marcel Proust, suggests that "the creation of the world did not take place in one day, but takes place every day."[2] The observation is completely unambiguous when read through the lives of the young men and women I followed. Moreover, the way one *senses* the world in Proust's novels, through memory, its objects, and its *reassignment* in the present, retains its force in the lifeworlds in which these young men and women participate. The present is inhabited and interpreted—formed, deformed, and created every day. Reflecting back on the first conversations I had with Jeff soon after he returned from detoxification, I remember how reluctant he was to describe his experiences with opiate withdrawal. "You have to be there" was an expression that challenged me and at the same time indicated that words fail because they were, in a sense, out of time. It was not that the experience defied language, but that the language found in the pain, discomfort, and euphoria he felt required "being there" to situate his words.[3] Over days and weeks, somehow he slowly became convinced that "being there" and feeling something firsthand were not the same things. "I'm right *here* motherfucker. Deal with it," was a favorite turn of phrase that Jeff used, often accompanied with several pumps of his fist on his chest. I liked the expression, not just because it was provocative (though there was that), but also because I was trying to do precisely what he was suggesting—to *deal* with Jeff's presence. Over time, the threat of "thinking somebody understands" receded from Jeff's concerns. "Even if you was standing right next to me, you asking me questions, you'd have no idea," he explained.

Later, after he had so lucidly given words to his experience of withdrawal, Jeff told me that he had to relive the experience a little each time he thought about it. His descriptions could stand on their own in the sense that they did not require a constant reference to his past experience, but it was into his past that he would continually reach. The last conversation we had together, several weeks before his death, was revealing. He spoke strongly about forgetting his past, disconnecting entirely from it. He was angry and regretful and it showed. My presence, my "being there," as someone who continually reminded him of a past that he wanted and needed to extinguish, proved too much to tolerate. Our conversations only "dredged shit up." Jeff's *past* life of drug dependence needed distancing from his *present* life of selling drugs illicitly on the street. If this distance was to be maintained, I could no longer spend time with him.

The career of a therapy does not just happen in the wake of medical intervention, but is how therapy is borne out. The idea I've tried to deal with is the concept of an *afterlife* of therapeutics. The meaning, however, may not always be entirely transparent. The afterlife of a pharmacotherapy is very much fixed in the present. My attention *to what comes after a therapy*, after the criteria used to measure outcomes in a research study are exhausted, cannot help but remain in the present, even in times when things are either recalled from the past or are projected onto a future. I insist that the afterlife of a therapy is lived every day, forming and deforming the experience of a therapy, assigning and reassigning meaning. Beckett writes, "There is no escape from the hours and the days. There is no escape from yesterday because yesterday has deformed us, or been deformed by us."[4] The way yesterday comes to form and deform the present is not a given. It is (and has to be) made and newly inhabited every day. It is in this way that *success* and *failure* are dangerous claims in relation to drug dependency. *Cure* one day cannot suffer *un-cure* the next. So why was success so important and mean-ingful for the individuals with whom I talked, but was defined (and demon-strated) so differently in each case? Perhaps it is too much to accept the idea that the trajectory of a treatment can vary so uncontrollably, never reaching an end. Perhaps it is because the stakes ultimately remain so ambiguous, and the terms of success are transformed so radically from one moment to the next. In this way, any finitude is welcome. To really *know* if buprenorphine is a successful pharmacotherapy, in the long term, may also be too much to ask. The claim of success would require both a fixed window in time and a backward glance through this window, after all is said and done. Research science *does* provide such a window in the form of a clinical trial.[5] Yet with the experience of addiction and recovery, so much is obscured beyond this frame. Today always contains the potential to unmake yesterday and tomor-row when it comes to drug abuse, for better or worse. What we can (and do) know is that pharmacotherapy takes up residence in the lives of the adolescents under treatment, they dwell with it, and it directly shapes their experience of drug dependency. The promise of recovery offered through pharmacotherapy is folded again and again into the lifeworlds of those under treatment, even in the absence of a defining outcome.

In the end I have tried to resist the temptation of blithely assigning mean-ing to the lives of the young men and women I was fortunate enough to come to know. I have attempted to avoid theorizing the purchase drug dependency and its treatment have in each of their lives. Instead, I have undertaken the often delicate, always messy task of showing how the lives of these young men and women guide and assign value, meaning, and worth to pharma-ceutical intervention, in whatever form these things care to take. I say all of this knowing it, too, runs the risk of failure.

Notes

Introduction

The chapter epigraph is from Friedrich Nietzsche, *The Gay Science*, trans. Walter Kaufmann (New York: Random House, 1974), no. 120, 176–77.

1   The research was conducted under a training fellowship from the National Institutes of Health/National Institute on Drug Abuse (F31-0202039–Sponsor: Dr. Jonathan Ellen, Johns Hopkins University, School of Medicine, Department of Pediatrics). The Homewood Institutional Review Board of the Johns Hopkins University approved the research (HIRB No. 2006021 "Therapeutic Contexts for Substance Abusing Adolescents"). The names of the informants are pseudonyms.

2   Pronounced *byoo-pre-NOR-feen*.

3   Henry Spiller et al., "Epidemiological Trends in Abuse and Misuse of Prescription Opioids," *Journal of Addictive Diseases* 28, no. 2 (2009): 130–36; In addition, see Philippe Bourgois and Jeffery Schonberg, *Righteous Dopefiend* (Berkeley: University of California Press, 2009); and Nancy Campbell, *Discovering Addiction: The Science and Politics of Substance Abuse Research* (Ann Arbor: University of Michigan Press, 2007).

4   Because the adolescents I followed—even with a small group—varied so widely in terms of initiation and patterns of drug use during their albeit short careers, it becomes impossible to talk about a general, meaningful "adolescent experience of drug abuse." Such a phrase would be completely empty. This, however, is not to imply that these adolescents did not exhibit some very broad "patterns" of use and abuse. The point I am attempting to make is that individual patterns are more productive if one wishes to understand the impact of treatment *on individuals*, which demands the avoidance of generalizations or hollow categorizations.

5   In terms of therapeutic and experimental bodies, I'm thinking specifically of Adriana Petryna's work on the utilization of human subjects for randomized controlled trials, "Ethical Variability: Drug Development and Globalizing Clinical Trials," *American Ethnologist* 32, no.2 (2005): 183–97. In the small group I fol-

lowed, two of the adolescents died—one as the result of an overdose, and one in a drug-related shooting. The notion of "shadow" here draws directly on Annette Leibing's work in *Shadow Side: Exploring the Blurred Borders Between Ethnography and Life*, ed. Athena McLean and Annette Leibing (Oxford: Blackwell Publishing, 2007).

6   Throughout this book I use the term "adolescents." From a certain perspective this is correct, at least in terms of their developmental stage and how they were regarded institutionally. However, I followed these adolescents for several years, and during that time they moved (developmentally and otherwise) from adolescence to young adulthood—not to mention that, because of their circumstances, many of them had "aged" well beyond their years. I've retained the term "adolescents" to distinguish them from adults, to avoid confusion by moving between terms, and to keep the focus centered on the institutional and clinical situations in which they found themselves. When I slip out of this nomenclature it has more to do with a stylistic choice than a theoretical one.

7   I use the term "following" in order to contrast "leading," as in "leading one to cure." But "tracing" is equally appropriate here, because I suggest that my ethnographic descriptions provide only contour lines around the adolescents I attempted to follow.

8   Roma Chatterji, "An Ethnography of Dementia," *Culture, Medicine, and Psychiatry* 22, no. 3 (1988): 355–82.

9   Buprenorphine was discovered in 1966. In 1975, Donald Jasinski began a small clinical trial using Buprenex (an analgesic licensed for the treatment of moderate to severe pain) in an attempt to treat opiate dependence in adults addicted to heroin. Jasinski and his colleagues conducted their work at the Bayview Hospital in Baltimore, one of the Johns Hopkins University medical centers. A series of randomized controlled trials followed, comparing the efficacy of buprenorphine (a partial μ-receptor agonist) against methadone (a full μ-receptor agonist). At that time there were also a number of trials comparing buprenorphine to placebo-controlled groups. As part of the Federal Drug Addiction Treatment Act (DATA) in 2000, buprenorphine was rescheduled by the Drug Enforcement Administration (DEA), which allowed physicians to prescribe the drug privately (albeit in regulated fashion) rather than in monitored settings such as methadone clinics. The FDA approved two new drugs for use in opiate dependency treatment, Subutex and Suboxone, in 2002. I describe these historical points in detail in chapter 1. See Nancy Campbell and Anne M. Lovell, "The History of the Development of Buprenorphine as an Addiction Therapeutic," *Annals of the New York Academy of Sciences* 1248 (2012): 124–39.

10   See Harry Marks's invaluable book, *The Progress of Experiment: Science and Therapeutic Reform in the United States, 1900–1990* (New York: Cambridge University Press, 1997); see also R. J. Matthews, *Quantification and the Quest for Medical Certainty* (Princeton, NJ: Princeton University Press, 1995).

11   Adriana Petryna, *When Experiments Travel: Clinical Trials and the Global Search for Human Subjects* (Princeton, NJ: Princeton University Press, 2009); see also Steven Epstein, *Inclusion: The Politics of Difference in Medical Research* (Chicago: University of Chicago Press, 2007).

12   Campbell, *Discovering Addiction*, 12–28; see also Robert Castel, *La gestion des risques* (Paris: Les Editions du Minuit, 1981). Janis Jenkins has recently described such lasting dilemmas of treatment as "recovery *without* cure" and "stigma *despite* recovery," in *Pharmaceutical Self: The Global Shaping of Experience in an Age of Psychopharmacology*, ed. Janis H. Jenkins (Santa Fe, NM: School for Advanced Research Press, 2012), 9.

13   See Jacques Derrida, *Archive Fever*, trans. Eric Prenowitz (Chicago: University of Chicago Press, 1995). I am approaching the idea of "the archive" (*arkhé*) in the way Derrida suggests, as a spatialized act where *thoughts* and *objects* are "commenced."

14   I use the phrase "a history of the present" along the lines Michel Foucault suggests in his *Discipline and Punish: The Birth of the Prison*, trans. A. Sheridan (New York: Vintage, 1977); see also Campbell and Lovell, "History and Development of Buprenorphine," 132.

15   See Ilana Löwy's preface to the French translation of Ludwik Fleck's *Genèse et développement d'un fait scientifique* (Paris: Flammarion, 2008).

16   In *Of Prognosis* (168 AD), Galen describes medical treatment as move way from individual healing through a change in the expectations (events) held by patients to those held by healers. Along a similar line of thought, writings in the Hippocratic canon are firm in their suggestion that healing, like symptoms, depends solely on the individual—that is to say, healing and illness are individual expressions. See specifically Michel Foucault's discussion of medical humanism in his "Preface" to *The Birth of the Clinic*, trans. A. Sheridan (New York: Vintage, 1973).

17   Georges Canguilhem, *Writings on Medicine*, trans. Stefanos Geroulanos and Todd Meyers (New York: Fordham University Press, 2012), 53–66.

18   As in the French *guérir*. Here there is the possibility of confusion between old and new terms, with the older term (after Alain Rey, *Dictionnaire de la langue française*) being "defender, protéger." The main definition is "protéger, garantir," and in this sense the proper term is "to defend." To "guard against" is another example, with the word *guérite*, from *guarir* or *garir*, "protéger." The modern terms, *protection* and *security*, still refer to the political assertions of public health from the nineteenth and twentieth centuries in France. The point is that there is a certain caution against anachronisms in etymology. See my introduction to Canguilhem's *Writings on Medicine* (with Stefanos Geroulanos), "Georges Canguilhem's Critique of Medical Reason," 1–24.

19   For a reading of Canguilhem's formulations in relation to the thought of Nietzsche, Levinas, and others, see in particular chapters 3 and 4 of Roberto

Esposito's *Bíos: Biopolitics and Philosophy*, trans. Timothy Campbell (Minneapolis, MN: University of Minnesota Press, 2008).

20 See Canguilhem, "Qu'est-ce que la psychologie," in *Études d'histoire et de philosophie des sciences* (Paris: J. Vrin, 1968), 367.

21 Canguilhem, *Writings on Medicine*, 55.

22 Georges Canguilhem, *The Normal and the Pathological*, trans. C. Fawcett (New York: Zone Books, 1989), 91.

23 Nowhere has the problem been more apparent than in debates regarding anti-retroviral therapy adherence in the context of HIV treatment. See João Biehl, *Will to Live: AIDS Therapies and the Politics of Survival* (Princeton, NJ: Princeton University Press, 2007); see also Lori Leonard's work with adolescents in the United States in Lori Leonard and Jonathan Ellen, "'The Story of My Life': AIDS and Autobiographical Occasions," *Qualitative Sociology* 31, no. 1 (2008): 37–56.

24 Jeremy Greene has demonstrated the point elegantly. See Jeremy A. Greene, "Therapeutic Infidelities: Noncompliance Enters the Medical Literature: 1955–1975," *Social History of Medicine* 17, no. 3 (2004): 327–43; see also Jeremy A. Greene, *Prescribing by Numbers: Drugs and the Definition of Disease* (Baltimore, MD: Johns Hopkins University Press, 2007).

25 Canguilhem, *Writings on Medicine*, 34–42.

26 Georges Canguilhem, "The Normal and the Pathological," in *Knowledge of Life*, ed. Paola Marrati and Todd Meyers, trans. Stefanos Geroulanos and Daniela Ginsburg (New York: Fordham University Press, 2008), 121–33.

27 Canguilhem, *Writings on Medicine*, 43–52.

28 Canguilhem, *The Normal and the Pathological*, 127. For a discussion of the reliance on statistical norms in the creation of public health and collective medical administrations, see Michel Foucault's essay, "The Birth of Social Medicine," in *The Essential Works of Foucault, 1954–1984, Vol. III, Power*, trans. R. Hurley (New York: The New Press, 2000).

29 Virginia Woolf, *On Being Ill* (New York: Paris Press, 2002), 7. Woolf writes, "The merest schoolgirl, when she falls in love, has Shakespeare or Keats to speak her mind for her; but let a sufferer try to describe a pain in his head to a doctor and language at once runs dry."

30 Canguilhem, *The Normal and the Pathological*, 115.

31 See Erving Goffman's later work, *Forms of Talk* (Philadelphia: University of Pennsylvania Press, 1981).

32 Arthur Kleinman, *The Illness Narratives: Suffering, Healing, and the Human Condition* (New York: Basic Books, 1987). For a discussion of how symptomatology and subjectivity are together borne out in anthropological theory, see João Biehl's essay (with Amy Moran-Thomas), "Symptom: Subjectivities, Social Ills, Technologies," *Annual Review of Anthropology* 38 (2009): 267–88.

33 Kleinman, *The Illness Narratives*, 5.

34 Ibid., 14.

35   In a short essay on chronic illness and dying, "A Turn Towards Dying: Presence, Signature, and the Social Course of Chronic Illness in Urban America,"
Medical Anthropology 26 (2007): 205–27, I refer to the "character" of speech in the
ethnography of illness as meeting somewhere in the middle of what Stefania
Pandolfo takes from Gilles Deleuze as a *double becoming.* She writes, "The author
takes a step towards his characters, but the characters take a step towards the
authors: *double becoming.* Storytelling (*la fabulation*) is not an impersonal myth,
but neither is it a personal fiction: in is *parole en acte*, a speech act through which
the character keeps crossing the boundary which would separate his private
business from politics, and himself produces collective utterances." *Impasse of
the Angels: Scenes from a Moroccan Space of Memory* (Chicago: University of Chicago
Press, 1997), 312–13.

36   Clifford Geertz, *The Interpretation of Cultures* (New York: Basic Books, 1973), 13.

37   For an important discussion of historical and epistemological perspectives, see
François Delaporte's "Foucault, Canguilhem et les monstres," in *Canguilhem, histoire des sciences et politique du vivant*, ed. Jean-François Braunstein (Paris: Presses
Universitaires de France, 2007). See also Michel Foucault, *The Birth of the Clinic*,
for a methodological demonstration of what it means to fold the absent into the
founding of the new (the clinical gaze). On the question of "silence" (or at least
the absence of narration), see Stanley Cavell's brief but provocative introduction
to a book on the making of Robert Gardner's film *Forest of Bliss*. Cavell writes,
"The absence of words magnified my own silence, or say, it called my silence
into question." See Gardner's *Making Forest of Bliss: Intention, Circumstance, and
Chance in Nonfiction Film* (Cambridge, MA: Harvard Film Archive, 2001), 9.

38   See Gérard Jorland and George Weisz, "Introduction: Who Counts?" in *Body
Counts: Medical Quantification in Historical and Sociological Perspectives*, ed. G.
Jorland, A. Opinel, and G. Weisz (Montreal: McGill-Queen's University Press,
2005), 3.

39   For a discussion of the aftermath of medical failure and what this failure says
about the anticipation and expectations of therapeutic practice—in his account,
specifically between local medical practices and western medical intervention
in Papua New Guinea—see Gilbert Lewis's *A Failure of Treatment* (New York:
Oxford University Press, 2000).

40   For a discussion of the reshaping of medical practice in relation to patient care
and clinical epidemiology, see Jeanne Daly's *Evidence-Based Medicine and the
Search for a Science of Clinical Care* (Berkeley: University of California Press, 2005).

41   Kurt Goldstein, *The Organism* (New York: Zone Books, 1995).

42   Gilles Deleuze, *Pure Immanence: Essays on A Life*, trans. Anne Boyman (New York:
Zone Books, 2001), 58.

43   Canguilhem tells us that authors as different as Henri Laugier, Henry Siger-
ist, and Kurt Goldstein each shared a perspective: "we cannot determine the
normal by simple reference to a statistical mean but only by comparing the indi-

vidual to itself, either in identical successive situations or in varied situations."
Canguilhem, *Knowledge of Life*, 129. For instance, Goldstein does not abandon the
diagnostic category, but is focused on how the individual inhabits and remakes
the category itself.

Firstly, I need to be clear when I say that the individual has the potential
to unmake what is known about the collective when delving into the question
of addiction, and perhaps disorder more generally. I'm not at all arguing for a
totalizing individualism in medical science. I'm not trying to replace univer-
salisms with particularisms. Secondly, there is a fine literature on the adolescent brain in relation to addiction, both in its distinction from the adult brain
(developmentally) and in the special risks involved with exposing *this* brain to
drugs of any kind. See T. L. Jernigan et al., "Maturation of Human Cerebrum
Observed in vivo During Adolescence," *Brain* 114 (1991): 2037–49; see also R. E.
Dahl and L. P. Spear, eds., "Adolescent Brain Development: Vulnerabilities and
Opportunities," *Annals of the New York Academy of Sciences* 1021 (2004): 1–469. I am
simply arguing for a finer brush to portray and understand the lives of adolescents who abuse drugs, one where the individual is not subject to abstraction.

44 I thank François Delaporte for providing his insight regarding these details.
Also see my introduction (with Stefanos Geroulanos) to Georges Canguilhem's
Writings on Medicine, 23–24.

45 I am referring to the Latin, *testimonium*, with its theological implications: *Deus
est fides, veritas est testimonium* "God is faith, truth is evidence." In the work of
Michel Foucault, in his third volume of *History of Sexuality*, we find the con-
nections between saying and knowing (confession)—as well as concealment—
regarded as components that shape self-knowledge.

46 Michel Foucault, *Dits et écrits, 1954–1975* (Paris: Gallimard, 1978), 540–41. I am
indebted to Sandra Laugier for drawing my attention to the passage.

47 The phrase "to dwell with the pain of withdrawal" requires a note of thanks to
Robert Desjarlais for offering his formulation.

48 See Nikolas Rose, *The Politics of Life Itself: Biomedicine, Power, and Subjectivity in the
Twenty-First Century* (Princeton, NJ: Princeton University Press, 2006); Andrew
Lakoff, *Pharmaceutical Reason: Knowledge and Value in Global Psychiatry* (New York:
Cambridge University Press, 2006); and the essays in Adriana Petryna, Andrew
Lakoff, Arthur Kleinman, eds., *Global Pharmaceuticals: Ethics, Markets, Practices*
(Durham, NC: Duke University Press, 2006).

49 See David Courtwright, *Dark Paradise: A History of Opiate Addiction in America*
(Cambridge, MA: Harvard University Press, 2001); Jill Jones, *Hep-Cats, Narcs,
and Pipe Dreams: A History of America's Romance with Illegal Drugs* (Baltimore, MD:
Johns Hopkins University Press, 1999).

50 On therapy and clinical reasoning in relation to biology, see François Dagognet's
La raison et les remèdes (Paris: Presses Universitaires de France, 1964).

51 Canguilhem, *Writings on Medicine*, 66.

1 / New Uses for Old Things

1   David A. Fiellin, "The First Three Years of Buprenorphine in the United States: Experience to Date and Future Directions," *Journal of Addiction Medicine* 1, no. 2 (2007): 62–67; see also J. M. Tetrault and D. A. Fiellin, "Current and Potential Pharmacological Treatment Options for Maintenance Therapy in Opioid-Dependent Individuals," *Drugs* 72, no. 2 (2012): 217–28.

2   Reckitt Benckiser Pharmaceuticals, "Reckitt Benckiser Pharmaceuticals Inc. Receives FDA Approval for Suboxone® (Buprenorphine and Naloxone) Sublingual Film C-III" (press release, August 31, 2010).

3   T. R. Kosten, C. Morgan, and H. O. Kleber, "Phase II Clinical Trials of Buprenorphine: Detoxification and Induction onto Naltrexone," *NIDA Monograph* 121 (1992): 101–19; J. W. Lewis and D. Walter, "Buprenorphine—Background to Its Development as a Treatment for Opiate Dependence," *NIDA Monograph* 21 (1992): 5–11.

4   L. Gowing and A. White, "Buprenorphine for the Management of Opioid Dependence: Review," *Cochrane Database of Systematic Reviews* 2, no. 3 (2006): CD002025.

5   Ibid.

6   N. D. Volkow, "What Do We Know about Drug Addiction?" *American Journal of Psychiatry* 162 (2005): 1401–2.

7   João Biehl, *Will to Live: AIDS Therapies and the Politics of Survival* (Princeton, NJ: Princeton University Press, 2009).

8   Vinh-Kim Nguyen, *The Republic of Therapy: Triage and Sovereignty in West Africa's Time of AIDS* (Durham, NC: Duke University Press, 2010).

9   Adriana Petryna, *When Experiments Travel: Clinical Trials and the Global Search for Human Subjects* (Princeton, NJ: Princeton University Press, 2009).

10 Andrew Lakoff, *Pharmaceutical Reason: Knowledge and Value in Global Psychiatry* (New York: Cambridge University Press, 2005).

11 Angela Garcia, *The Pastoral Clinic: Addiction and Dispossession Along the Rio Grande* (Berkeley: University of California Press, 2010).

12 M. Fishman, A. Bruner, and H. Adger, "Substance Abuse among Children and Adolescents," *Pediatric Review* 18 (1997): 394–403.

13 Maurice Merleau-Ponty, *The Visible and the Invisible*, trans. Alphonso Lingis (Evanston, IL: Northwestern University Press, 1968).

14 Michael Taussig, *I Swear I Saw This: Drawings in Fieldwork Notebooks, Namely My Own* (Chicago: University of Chicago Press, 2011), xi.

15 George E. Woody, Sabrina A. Poole, Geetha Subramaniam, et al., "Extended vs. Short-term Buprenorphine-Naloxone for Treatment of Opioid-Addicted Youth: A Randomized Trial," *Journal of the American Medical Association* 300, no.17 (2008): 2003–11. The outline of the protocol and the outcomes are derived from Woody et al. (2008) and the Clinical Trials Network protocol website:

http://clinicaltrials.gov/ct2/show/NCT00078130 (accessed 29 November 2008).

16 Ibid.

17 Carl Levin, "FDA Approval of Buprenorphine" and "FDA Approval of Medication to Combat Heroin Addiction Culminates Long-Fought Battle, Says Levin" (press releases, October 9, 2002).

18 United States House of Representatives, *Drug Addiction Treatment Act of 1999: Report Together with Additional Views (to accompany H.R. 2634; including cost estimate of the Congressional Budget Office)* (Washington, DC: Government Printing Office, 1999). Included in the testimony is a letter from Representative John D. Dingell, which speaks directly to the issue of new groups of users: "buprenorphine and buprenorphine/naloxone products are expected to reach new groups of opiate addicts—for example, those who do not have access to methadone programs, those who are reluctant to enter methadone programs, and those who are unsuited to them (this would include, for example, those in their first year of opiate addiction or those addicted to lower doses of opiates)."

19 Carl Levin (press release), October 9, 2002.

20 D. R. Jasinski, J. S. Pevnick, and J. D. Griffith, "Human pharmacology and Abuse Potential of the Analgesic Buprenorphine: A Potential Agent for Treating Narcotic Addiction," *Archives of General Psychiatry* 35, no. 4 (1978): 501–16. Coincidentally, 1978 is the same year that Georges Canguilhem published "Is a Pedagogy of Healing Possible?"

21 Lindsey Jorgensen provided additional details during conversations while profiling buprenorphine for the Project Impact Study at the Johns Hopkins School of Medicine (Steven Goodman and Harry Marks, principle investigators).

22 Walter Ling and Donald R. Wesson, "Clinical Efficacy of Buprenorphine: Comparisons to Methadone and Placebo," *Drug and Alcohol Dependence* 70 (2003): S49–S57; Warren K. Bickel et al., "A Clinical Trial of Buprenorphine: Comparison with Methadone in the Detoxification of Heroin Addicts," *Clinical Pharmacology & Therapeutics* 43, no. 1 (1988): 72–78.

23 Rolley E. Johnson, Thomas Eissenberg, et al., "A Placebo Controlled Clinical Trial of Buprenorphine as a Treatment for Opioid Dependence," *Drug and Alcohol Dependence* 40 (1995): 17–25; Rolley E. Johnson, Jerome H. Jaffe, and Paul J. Fudala, "A Controlled Trial of Buprenorphine Treatment for Opioid Dependence," *Journal of the American Medical Association* 267, no. 20 (1992): 2750–55.
    While these trials began in 1992, it is important to note that the French began office-based treatment with buprenorphine in 1996, once significant questions were answered about side effects, dose response, and concerns with outcomes like respiratory depression, with Subutex—high-dose buprenorphine—and while the drug was only licensed to treat pain, off-label prescribing began widely in 1996. In 1997, Schering Plough Corporation entered a fifteen-year worldwide rights agreement with Reckitt Benckiser to distribute buprenorphine globally. Schering Plough merged with Merck & Co. in 2009. See Anne M.

Lovell, "Addiction Markets: The Case of High-dose Buprenorphine in France," in *Global Pharmaceuticals*, ed. A. Petryna et al. (2006); see also Nancy Campbell and Anne M. Lovell, "The History of the Development of Buprenorphine as an Addiction Therapeutic," *Annals of the New York Academy of Sciences* 1248 (2012): 124–39.

24 Food and Drug Administration, "Drug Shortage: Drug to be Discontinued Letter from Roxane (ORLAAM [Levomethadyl hydrochloride acetate] Solution)" (press release, August 23, 2003).

25 Herbert D. Kleber, "Naltrexone," *Journal of Substance Abuse Treatment* 2 (1985): 117–22.

26 Warren K. Bickel et al., "A Clinical Trial of Buprenorphine," 72–78.

27 Rolley E. Johnson, Edward J. Cone, et al., "Use of Buprenorphine in the Treatment of Opiate Addiction: I. Physiologic and Behavioral Effects During a Rapid Dose Induction," *Clinical Pharmacology & Therapeutics* 46, no. 3 (1989): 335–43; Paul J. Fudala et al., "Use of Buprenorphine in the Treatment of Opioid Addiction: II. Physiologic and Behavioral Effects of Daily and Alternate-day Administration and Abrupt Withdrawal," *Clinical Pharmacology & Therapeutics* 47, no. 4 (1990): 525–34.

28 Alan Cowan and John W. Lewis, eds., *Buprenorphine: Combating Drug Abuse with a Unique Opioid* (New York: Wiley-Liss Publications, 1995).

29 John W. Lewis and Donald Walter, "Buprenorphine—Background to Its Development"; Thomas R. Kosten, Charles Morgan, and Herbert O. Kleber, "Phase II Clinical Trials of Buprenorphine," NIDA Monograph 21 (1992):5-11."

30 Katharine P. Bailey, "Pharmacological Treatments for Substance Use Disorders," *Journal of Psychosocial Nursing* 42, no. 8 (2004): 14–20.

31 Mary Jeanne Kreek, "Methadone-Related Opioid Agonist Pharmacotherapy for Heroin Addiction: History, Recent Molecular and Neuro-chemical Research and Future in Mainstream Medicine," *Annals of the New York Academy of Sciences* 909 (2000): 186–216.

32 Mark B. McClellan, "Two Drugs for Opioid Dependence," *Journal of the American Medical Association* 288, no. 21 (2002): 2678.

33 Federal Register, "Buprenorphine Prescribing Practices Survey," 67, no. 233 (2002): 72219; Federal Register, "Meeting on Buprenorphine Treatment," 67, no. 175 (2002): 57445.

34 On October 17, 2000, President Bill Clinton signed into law the Drug Addiction Treatment Act of 2000 (DATA), Title XXXV, Section 3502 of the Children's Health Act of 2000. DATA expanded the context of medication-assisted treatment by allowing qualified physicians to prescribe or dispense approved Schedule III, IV, and V medications for detoxification and maintenance treatment of dependency. In addition, DATA reduced the regulatory burden on physicians by permitting them to apply for and receive waivers from the special registration requirements defined in the Federal Controlled Substances Act.

35 The Controlled Substances Act was part of the 1970 congressional reform.

Schedule V drugs include those containing opiates, and schedule IV drugs include long-acting barbiturates and non-amphetamine stimulants.

36 The Orphan Drug Act passed into law in January 1983. The two drugs developed by Reckitt Benckiser received orphan drug status in 1994.

37 See Highlights of Recent Reports on Substance Abuse and Mental Health, U.S. Department of Health and Human Services, Substance Abuse and Mental Health Services Administration, Office of Applied Studies, http://www.oas. samhsa.gov/highlights.htm (accessed 10 October 2008).

38 L. D. Johnston, P. M. O'Malley, J. G. Bachman, and J. E. Schulenberg, *Monitoring the Future National Survey Results on Drug Use, 1975–2007, Vol. I, Secondary School Students*, NIH Publication No. 08-6418A (Bethesda, MD: National Institute on Drug Abuse, 2007).

39 Ibid.; the increases were also reported in an editorial by David A. Fiellin, "Treatment of Adolescent Opioid Dependence: No Quick Fix," *Journal of the American Medical Association* 300, no. 17 (2008): 2057–59.

40 John M. Wallace Jr. and Jerald G. Bachman, "Explaining Racial/Ethnic Differences in Adolescent Drug Use: The Impact of Background and Lifestyle," *Social Problems* 38, no. 3 (1991): 333–57.

41 Nancy Campbell and Susan Shaw, "Incitements to Discourse: Illicit Drugs, Harm Reduction, and the Production of Ethnographic Subjects," *Cultural Anthropology* 23, no. 4 (2009): 688–717; see also Angela Garcia's *The Pastoral Clinic* on heroin use in family networks.

42 Fiellin, "Treatment of Adolescent Opioid Dependence," 2057–59.

43 David A. Fiellin, "The First Three Years of Buprenorphine in the United States," 62–67.

44 N. D. Volkow, "What Do We Know about Drug Addiction?" 1401–02.

45 B. Lopez et al., "Adolescent Neurological Development and Its Implications for Adolescent Substance Abuse Prevention," *Journal of Primary Prevention* 29, no. 1 (2008): 5–35.

46 See Carl Levin, Congressional Record—Senate, and Commentaries, S1091–S1093, January 28, 1999.

47 The trial examined the transition to naltrexone in patients receiving buprenorphine versus clonidine, cited in L. A. Marsch, W. K. Bickel, G. J. Badger, M. E. Stothart, et al., "Comparison of Pharmacological Treatments for Opioid-Dependent Adolescents," *Archives of General Psychiatry* 62, no. 10 (2005): 1157–64.

48 Ibid.

49 P. A. Donaher and C. Welsh, "Managing Opioid Addiction with Buprenorphine: Review." *American Family Physician* 73, no. 9 (2006): 1573–78.

50 For a review of the neuro-biological effects of treatment in the long-term, see T. R. Kosten and T. P. George, "The Neurobiology of Opioid Dependence: Implications for Treatment," *Science & Practice Perspectives* 1, no. 1 (2002): 13–20. For a

review of the psychosocial components of long-term treatment, see L. Amato et al., "Psychosocial and Pharmacological Treatments versus Pharmacological Treatments for Opioid Detoxification." *Cochrane Database Systematic Reviews* 3 (2008): CD005031.

51 Food and Drug Administration, "Subutex and Suboxone Approved to Treat Opiate Dependence" (press release, October 2, 2002).

52 Directly observed therapy has been the standard of care in the treatment of tuberculosis since 1993; see Ronald Bayer and David Wilkinson, "Directly Observed Therapy for Tuberculosis: History of an Idea," *Lancet* 345, no. 8964 (1995): 1545. Directly observed therapy has also recently moved into antiretroviral drug therapy; see Paul Farmer et al., "Letter to the Editor: Directly Observed Therapy for HIV Anti-retroviral Therapy in an Urban U.S. Setting," *Journal of Acquired Immune Deficiencies Syndrome* 36, no. 91 (2004): 642–44.

53 Mary Jeanne Kreek and Frank J. Vocci, "History and Current Status of Opioid Maintenance Treatments: Blending Conference Session," *Journal of Substance Abuse Treatment* 23 (2002): 93–105.

54 J. Gaertner, R. Voltz, and C. Ostgathe, "Methadone: A Closer Look at the Controversy," *Journal of Pain Symptom Management* 36, no. 2 (2008): e4–e7.

55 The grand round focused specifically on peer-to-peer HIV counseling in one of the hospital's clinics. The presentation was given jointly by a physician and a patient who had become a peer counselor.

56 Anna Ditkoff, "Bloodletting: Can Anything Be Done to Bring Baltimore's Homicide Rate Down?" *The City Paper*, January 23, 2008.

57 Todd Meyers, Lori Leonard, and Jonathan M. Ellen, "The Clinic and Elsewhere: Illness, Sexuality and Social Experience among Young African-American Men in Baltimore, Maryland," *Culture, Medicine, and Psychiatry* 289, no. 1 (2004): 67–86. See also Allan Brandt, "Behavior, Disease, and Health in the Twentieth-Century United States: The Moral Valence of Individual Risk," in *Morality and Health: Interdisciplinary Perspectives*, ed. A. Brandt and P. Rozin (New York: Routledge, 1997), 53–78.

58 I was later told the "sword" was meant to represent the staff carried by Hermes, to symbolize peace. However, it still looks like a sword—and patients complained that it made the pills hard to cut evenly.

59 Truesdell S. Brown, *Timaeus of Tauromenium* (Berkeley: University of California, 1958).

60 S. J. Becker and J. F. Curry, "Outpatient Interventions for Adolescent Substance Abuse: A Quality of Evidence Review," *Journal of Consulting and Clinical Psychology* 76, no. 4 (2008): 531–43.

61 H. D. Kleber, "Methadone Maintenance Four Decades Later: Thousands of Lives Saved but Still Controversial," *Journal of the American Medical Association* 300, no. 19 (2008): 2303–05.

2 / Monasticism

The epigraph is from Gaston Bachelard, *The Poetics of Space*, trans. M. Jolas (New York: Beacon Press, 1994), 47.

1   Anyone familiar with the field of substance-abuse treatment in Maryland will likely already know the residential treatment center where I conducted my research, and while permission to conduct my research in the treatment center was granted, I have chosen not to identify the treatment center by name in the book in order to retain whatever anonymity is possible. I do this for two reasons. First, I'd like to protect, in a small way, the clinicians, staff, and patients from being identified—or at least make it more difficult to put *names and faces* to *stories*. My writing is in no way meant to be an exposé, and it needs to be clear that the work the clinicians and staff do at the treatment center is tremendous—and tremendously difficult. Second, while the treatment center is indeed important as a locality, my argument is that, like a number of other clinical and nonclinical institutional environments, it is a space that affords highly porous relationships between the social worlds inside and outside its walls. To say this another way, I am not trying to simply offer an institutional history of the treatment center.

2   For a discussion of the types of speech and personhood that arise from therapeutic interactions, see E. Summerson Carr's *Scripting Addiction: The Politics of Therapeutic Talk and American Sobriety* (Princeton, NJ: Princeton University Press, 2010).

3   P. Clemmey, L. Payne, and M. Fishman, "Clinical Characteristics and Treatment Outcomes of Adolescent Heroin Users," *Journal of Psychoactive Drugs* 36 (2004): 85–94.

4   Ibid.; see also David Moshman, *Adolescent Rationality and Development: Cognition, Morality, Identity*, 3rd edition (New York: Psychology Press, 2011).

5   P. Clemmey, L. Payne, H. Adger, and M. Fishman, *Manual for a Short-Term Residential Treatment Program for Adolescent Substance Use Disorders* [title amended] (Bloomington, IL: Chestnut Health Systems, 2003).

6   Ibid.

7   Ibid.

8   Maurice Merleau-Ponty, *The Structure of Behavior*, trans. Alden L. Fisher (New York: Beacon Press, 1963), 62.

9   Michel Serres, *The Five Senses: The Philosophy of Mingled Bodies* (New York: Continuum Press, 2009), 3.

10   See the essay "58 Indices of the Body" in Jean-Luc Nancy, *Corpus*, trans. Richard Rand (New York: Fordham University Press, 2008), 150–60.

11   Allan Young, *The Harmony of Illusions: Inventing Post-Traumatic Stress Disorder* (Princeton, NJ: Princeton University Press, 1997).

12 See chapter 1 of this book; see also George E. Woody, Sabrina A. Poole, Geetha Subramaniam, et al., "Extended vs. Short-term Buprenorphine-Naloxone for Treatment of Opioid-Addicted Youth: A Randomized Trial," *Journal of the American Medical Association* 300, no. 17 (2008): 2003–11.

13 Kurt Goldstein, *The Organism* (New York: Zone Books, 2000), 30.

14 Ibid., 324.

15 Quoted widely by Georges Canguilhem; see the chapter "Health: Popular Concept and Philosophical Question" in *Writings on Medicine*, trans. Stefanos Geroulanos and Todd Meyers (New York: Fordham University Press, 2012).

16 Ibid.

17 Serres, *The Five Senses*, 85.

18 Ibid., 150.

19 Gilles Deleuze, *Francis Bacon: Logic of Sensation*, trans. Daniel W. Smith (Minneapolis: University of Minnesota Press, 2006).

20 See Daniel W. Smith's translator's introduction to Deleuze's *Francis Bacon*, "Deleuze on Bacon: Three Conceptual Trajectories in *The Logic of Sensation*," xiii.

21 Shigehisa Kuriyama, *The Expressiveness of the Body in Greek and Chinese Medicine* (New York: Zone Books, 2000).

22 Deleuze, *Francis Bacon*, 6.

23 Michel Foucault, *Dits et écrits, Tome 1, 1954–1975* (Paris: Gallimard, 1978), 540–41.

3 / Appropriations of Care

1 Annemarie Mol, *The Logic of Care: Health and the Problem of Patient Choice* (London: Routledge, 2008).

2 Ibid., 29

3 Ibid., 48–53

4 Arthur Frank, "Stories of Illness as Care of the Self: A Foucauldian Dialogue," *Health* 2 (1998): 329.

5 Michel Foucault, *The History of Sexuality, Vol. 3, The Care of the Self*, trans. Robert Hurley (New York: Pantheon, 1986); Michel Foucault, "Technologies of the Self," in *Technologies of the Self*, ed. L. H. Martin, H. Gutman, and P. H. Hutton (Amherst: University of Massachusetts Press, 1988), 16–49.

6 Sandra Laugier, "Wittgenstein and Cavell: Anthropology, Skepticism, and Politics," in *The Claim to Community: Essays on Stanley Cavell and Political Philosophy*, ed. Andrew Norris (Palo Alto, CA: Stanford University Press, 2006); Stanley Cavell, *Little Did I Know: Excerpts from Memory* (Palo Alto, CA: Stanford University Press, 2010); Pascale Molinier, Sandra Laugier, and Patricia Paperman, eds., *Qu'est-ce que le care?: Souci des autres, sensibilité, responsabilité* (Paris: Payot, 2009).

7 Carol Gilligan, *In a Different Voice: Psychological Theory and Women's Development* (Cambridge, MA: Harvard University Press, 1983); Vanessa Nurock, ed., *Carol Gilligan et l'éthique du care* (Paris: Presses Universitaires de France, 2010).

8   Michel Foucault, "The Ethics of the Concern for Self as a Practice of Freedom," in *The Essential Works of Foucault, 1954–1984, Vol. I, Ethics: Subjectivity and Truth*, ed. P. Rabinow (New York: The New Press, 1997), 281–302.

9   Marie Garrau and Alice Le Goff, *Care, justice, dépendance: Introduction aux théories du care* (Paris: Presses Universitaires de France, 2010); see also Frédéric Worms, *Le moment du soin* (Paris: Presses Universitaires de France, 2010), and Jean-Philippe Pierron, *Vulnérabilité: Pour une philosophie du soin* (Paris: Presses Universitaires de France, 2010).

10   Frédéric Worms, Céline Lefève, Lazare Benaroyo, and Jean-Christophe Mino, eds., *La philosophie du soin* (Paris: Presses Universitaires de France, 2010); see also Olivier Doron, Céline Lefève, and Alain-Charles Masquelet, eds., *Soin et subjectivité* (Paris: Presses Universitaires de France, 2010).

11   U.S. Department of Justice, Drug Enforcement Administration, Office of Diversion Control, "Schedule of Controlled Substances: Proposed Rule: Rescheduling Buprenorphine from Schedule V to Schedule III" (press release, March 21, 2002); National Institutes of Health, "Buprenorphine Approval Expands Options for Addiction Treatment," *National Institute on Drug Abuse Research News* 17, no. 4 (2002): 1.

12   Reckitt Benckiser Pharmaceuticals, "First New Addiction Treatment Products in 30 Years Approved for In-Office Treatment" (press release, October 9, 2002).

13   National Institutes of Health, "Hearing before the Health, Education, Labor, and Pensions Committee United States Senate: 'Oxycontin, Balancing Risks and Benefits'" (statement of record, February 12, 2002).

14   J. Gaertner, R. Voltz, and C. Ostgathe, "Methadone: A Closer Look at the Controversy." *Journal of Pain Symptom Management* 36, no. 2 (2008): e4-e7; A. G. Lipman, "Methadone: Effective Analgesia, Confusion, and Risk," *Journal of Pain and Palliative Care Pharmacotherapy* 19 (2005): 3–5.

15   Gaertner et al., "Methadone," e4.

16   The move toward de-specialization, at least in the case of addiction treatment, seems to run counter to the increase of specialization throughout the twentieth century described in George Weisz's important book, *Divide and Conquer: A Comparative History of Medical Specialization* (New York: Oxford University Press, 2006).

17   See B. R. Meier and A. A. Patkar, "Buprenorphine Treatment: Factors and First-Hand Experiences for Providers to Consider," *Journal of Addictive Diseases* 26, no. 1 (2007): 3–14; see also H. K. Knudsen, L. J. Ducharme, and P. M. Roman, "Early Adoption of Buprenorphine in Substance Abuse Treatment Centers: Data from the Private and Public Sectors," *Journal of Substance Abuse and Treatment* 30, no. 4 (2006): 363–73.

18   Jerome H. Jaffe and Charles O'Keeffe, "From Morphine Clinics to Buprenorphine: Regulating Opioid Agonist Treatment of Addiction in the United States," *Drug and Alcohol Dependence* 70 (2003): S3–S11.

19   Christopher S. Wren, "In Battle against Heroin, Scientists Enlist Heroin," *New*

York Times, June 8, 1999.

20 L. Amato, S. Minozzi, M. Davoli, S. Vecchi, M. M. Ferri, S. Mayet, "Psychosocial and Pharmacological Treatments versus Pharmacological Treatments for Opioid Detoxification," *Cochrane Database Systematic Reviews* 3 (2008): CD005031.

21 David A. Fiellin and Patrick G. O'Connor, "Office-Based Treatment of Opioid-Dependent Patients," *New England Journal of Medicine* 347 (2002): 817–23; John O'Neil, "Vital Signs: A New Drug Means a New Venue," *New York Times*, October 15, 2002; Richard Pérez-Peña, "New Drug Promises Shift in Treatment for Heroin Addicts," *New York Times*, August 11, 2003.

22 Sharon L. Walsh and Thomas Eissenberg, "The Clinical Pharmacology of Buprenorphine: Extrapolating from the Laboratory to the Clinic," *Drug and Alcohol Dependence* 70 (2003): S13–S27.

23 L. E. Sullivan and D. A. Fiellin, "Narrative Review: Buprenorphine for Opioid-Dependent Patients in Office Practice," *Annals of Internal Medicine* 148, no. 9 (2008): 662–70.

24 Ibid., 665.

25 Alison L. Koch, Cynthia L. Arfken, and Charles R. Schuster, "Characteristics of U.S. Substance Abuse Treatment Facilities Adopting Buprenorphine in Its Initial Stage of Availability," *Drug and Alcohol Dependence* 83, no. 3 (2006): 274–78.

26 For additional information on the use of methadone in primary care settings, see Patrick G. O'Connor et al., "A Randomized Trial of Buprenorphine Maintenance for Heroin Dependence in a Primary Care Clinic for Substance Users versus a Methadone Clinic," *American Journal of Medicine* 105 (1998): 100–105; Patrick G. O'Connor et al., "Three Methods of Opioid Detoxification in a Primary Care Setting: A Randomized Trial," *Annals of Internal Medicine* 127, no. 7 (1997): 526–30; Barbara J. Turner et al., "Barriers and Facilitators to Primary Care or Human Immunodeficiency Virus Clinics Providing Methadone or Buprenorphine for the Management of Opioid Dependence," *Archives of Internal Medicine* 165 (2005): 1769–76; Walter Ling, Leslie Amass, Steve Shoptaw, Jeffrey J. Annon, et al., "A Multi-Center Randomized Trial of Buprenorphine-Naloxone Versus Clonidine for Opioid Detoxification: Findings from the National Institute on Drug Abuse Clinical Trials Network," *Addiction* 100 (2005): 1090–1100.

27 For a review of treatment setting outcomes, see E. Day, J. Ison, and J. Strang, "Inpatient Versus Other Settings for Detoxification for Opioid Dependence," *Cochrane Database of Systematic Reviews* 2 (2005): CD004580.

28 David A. Fiellin, Robert A. Rosenheck, and Thomas R. Kosten, "Office-Based Treatment for Opioid Dependence: Reaching New Patient Populations," *American Journal of Psychiatry* 158 (2001): 1200–04.

29 Baltimore City Council President, "City Council President Stephanie Rawlings-Blake Calls for Public Hearing on Heroin Treatment: President to Request Expansion on City's Buprenorphine Availability" (press release, March 26, 2007).

30 Knudsen, "Early Adoption of Buprenorphine," 363.

31 Suzanne McMurphy et al., "Clinic-Based Treatment for Opioid Dependence: A Qualitative Inquiry," *American Journal of Health Behavior* 30, no. 6 (2006): 544–54.

4 / Therapy and Reason

1 Erika Niedowski, "Success, Setbacks in France, French Approach to Drug Offers Lessons that U.S. Has Largely Overlooked," *The Baltimore Sun*, December 17, 2007; Fred Schulte and Doug Donovan, "Drug Earning Millions Despite 'Orphan' Label: Status Granted Before Law Increased Use of 'Bupe,'" *The Baltimore Sun*, December 18, 2007; Doug Donovan and Fred Schulte, "Not a Cure-all: Despite Praise, 'Bupe' Alone Isn't Enough to Break Addicts of Destructive Routines," *The Baltimore Sun*, December 18, 2007.

2 Fred Schulte and Doug Donovan, "The 'Bupe' Fix, Promoted by the U.S. as a Treatment for Opiate Addiction: Buprenorphine Has Become One More Item for Sale in the Illegal Drug Market," *The Baltimore Sun*, December 16, 2007.

3 Rebecca Alvania, "Drug Disabuse: Bupe Treats Heroin Addiction Easily and Safely but Remains Hard to Come By," *The City Paper*, December 19, 2007.

4 The number of physicians does not include those working in treatment programs authorized under 21 U.S.C. Section 823 (g)(1) to dispense (but not prescribe) opioid treatment medications. Treatment programs registered under 21 U.S.C. Section 823 (g)(1) are not subject to patient limits.

5 In March 2008, I conducted a randomized phone survey with physicians (n = 126) in the Baltimore area who had received certification from SAMHSA after 2000 to prescribe buprenorphine. From the brief phone survey of eight questions, asked of those physicians who were currently prescribing Subutex or Suboxone on an outpatient basis (n = 86), none reported that they believed their patients were selling or distributing the drugs illegally, nor did they know of any reports (other than *The Baltimore Sun* articles, which were specifically referenced) of illegal distribution or sale. When I asked if the physicians believed their patients were abusing the drugs, in several cases the physicians asked, "You know how the drug works, right?" referring to the low abuse potential of Suboxone, given its dose response threshold. By *believe* I was interested in physicians' perceptions about abuse and diversion, rather than empirically identified cases.

6 Rolley E. Johnson, "Letter from Reckitt Benckiser VP for Scientific and Regulatory Affairs," *The Baltimore Sun*, December 17, 2007. Here is an excerpt of his statement:

> We are totally committed to reducing the harm of this devastating and misunderstood disease state, and to helping as many individuals as possible into successful, long-term treatment. To this end, we have worked closely with the government, the addiction medical societies, and key thought leaders in the field of addiction to bring this medical

treatment forward for the millions of everyday Americans who need treatment. . . . Our objective is for buprenorphine treatment to be a powerful intervention to what has become a public health threat. Certainly we as individuals and as a company are concerned about any possible misuse and/or diversion of our products, and from the beginning have worked to establish mechanisms that enable us to work with the government, law enforcement, and indeed the clinical community to curb the likelihood and extent of such illegal activity. . . . Additionally, the company has made and continues to make significant investments in creating an abuse-resistant distribution network. We also have and continue to maintain a proactive and open communication with our physician base to educate them as to their role in minimizing potential diversion and misuse. The company's extensive and ongoing additional financial investments were anticipated at the outset as part of the cost of doing business in a disease . . . that is as highly stigmatized and inherently risky as addiction treatment. Any treatment of this type will carry an additional corporate burden; the patient population is at higher risk of misuse and/or diversion by the very nature of their chronic medical condition, and one must have realistic expectations. But despite the risks, it is a testament to the value of this medical treatment that the vast majority of patients are receiving a safe and effective, FDA-approved treatment for a condition (and a social public health threat) that has defied so many previous attempts to overcome it.

7   In addition to problems with surveillance, Reckitt Benckiser acknowledged problems such as children sickened by accidentally ingesting pills in a report submitted to the FDA on January 8, 2008. See Cynthia G. McCormick et al., "Case Histories in Pharmaceutical Risk Management, *Drug and Alcohol Dependence* 105S (2009): S42-S55.

8   Joshua Sharfstein and Peter Luongo, "Addiction Poses Greater Dangers" (Letter to the editor), *The Baltimore Sun*, December 22, 2007.

9   H. S. Joseph, S. Stancliff, and J. Langrod, "Methadone Maintenance Treatment (MMT): A Review of Historical and Clinical Issues," *Mt. Sinai Journal of Medicine* 67, nos. 5-6 (2000): 347–64.

10   Center for a Healthy Maryland, "Report: Improving Patient Access to Buprenorphine Treatment through Physician Offices in Maryland," June 2007, http://www.healthymaryland.org/substance-use-buprenorphine.php (accessed 11 August 2007).

11   Fred Schulte and Doug Donovan, "Senators Urge Action to Reduce 'Bupe' Abuse, in MD: Lawmakers Vow Probe of State's Spending for Drug," *The Baltimore Sun*, December 20, 2007.

12   Fred Schulte and Doug Donovan, "Misuse of 'Bupe' Is Found to Be on the Rise,

Report Shows: U.S. Could Exert Controls if Problem Deemed Serious," *The Baltimore Sun*, February 3, 2008; Fred Schulte and Doug Donovan, "Agency Sat on 'Bupe' Study: Officials Waited to Reveal Findings on Misuse of Drug," *The Baltimore Sun*, February 12, 2008.

13 D. R. Jasinski, J. S. Pevnick, and J. D. Griffith, "Human Pharmacology and Abuse Potential of the Analgesic Buprenorphine," *Archives of General Psychiatry* 35, no. 4 (1978): 501–16.

14 Substance Abuse and Mental Health Service Administration, "Diversion and Abuse of Buprenorphine: A Brief Assessment of Emerging Indicators," December 2006. http://buprenorphine.samhsa.gov/Buprenorphine_FinalReport_12.6.06.pdf (accessed 2 July 2008).

15 Substance Abuse and Mental Health Service Administration, "Buprenorphine: Patient Limits Increase," *SAMHSA News* January/February (2007).

16 Charles R. Schuster, "Conversation with Charles R. Schuster," *Addiction* 99, no. 6 (2004): 667–76.

17 David A. Fiellin and Patrick G. O'Connor, "New Federal Initiatives to Enhance the Medical Treatment of Opioid Dependence," *Annals of Internal Medicine* 137, no. 8 (2002): 688–92.

18 R. E. Johnson, E. C. Strain, and L. Amass, "Review: Buprenorphine, How to Use It Right," *Drug and Alcohol Dependence* 70 (2003): S59–S77.

19 Fred Schulte and Doug Donovan, "Strategies to Control Bupe Abuse Outlined," *The Baltimore Sun*, February 23, 2008.

20 Doug Donovan and Fred Schulte, "Bupe Seizures Rise as Treatment Use Grows," *The Baltimore Sun*, April 18, 2008.

21 The quote in the article is drawn from a Center for Substance Abuse Treatment (SAMHSA/NIDA) workshop presentation, "Buprenorphine in the Treatment of Opioid Addiction: Expanding Access, Enhancing Quality," February 21–22, 2008, Washington, DC.

22 Christopher Welsh, "Addiction Poses Greater Dangers" (Letter to the editor), *The Baltimore Sun*, December 22, 2007.

23 Isabelle Feroni and Anne M. Lovell, "Les dispositifs de regulation publique d'un medicament sensible: Le cas du Subutex®, traitement de substitution aux opiaces," *Revue française des affaires sociales. Cahier de jurisprudence. Emploi-travail* 61, no. 3 (2007): 153–65.

24 Anne M. Lovell, "Addiction Markets: The Case of High-dose Buprenorphine in France," in *Global Pharmaceuticals*, ed. Adriana Petryna, Andrew Lakoff, and Arthur Kleinman (Durham, NC: Duke University Press, 2006).

25 Report of the Grand Jury for Baltimore City, January 7, 2008 through May 2, 2008; Baltimore Substance Abuse Systems, Inc., "The Baltimore Buprenorphine Initiative: Second Interim Progress Report," http://www.baltimorehealth.org/substanceabuse.html (accessed 2 December 2008).

26 Diana Morris, "Addiction Poses Greater Dangers" (Letter to the editor), *The Baltimore Sun*, December 22, 2007.

27 Anne M. Lovell, "Ordonner les risques: L'individu et le pharmaco-sociatif face à la réduction des dommages dans l'injection de drogues," in *Critique de la santé publique: Une approche anthropologique*, ed. Jean-Pierre Dozon and Didier Fassin (Paris: Balland, 2001).

28 Luc Boltanski, *La découverte de la maladie: La diffusion du savior medical* (Paris: Centre de sociologie européenne, 1968); Philippe Bourgois, "Intimate Apartheid: Ethnic dimensions of habitus among homeless heroin injectors," *Ethnography* 8, no. 1 (2007): 7–31. Regarding individual and familial experience in a different context, see Angela Garcia's excellent book, *The Pastoral Clinic*.

29 The concern with diversion continued to persist in the United States, with the same inattention to the patient–addict relationship, and with continued conflation of the two available forms of buprenorphine; see, for example, E. D. Wish et al., "The Emerging Buprenorphine Epidemic in the United States," *Journal of Addictive Diseases* 31, no. 1 (2012): 3–7.

30 D. H. Gandhi, G. J. Kavanagh, and J. H. Jaffe, "Young Heroin Users in Baltimore: A Qualitative Study," *American Journal of Drug and Alcohol Abuse* 32 (2006): 177–88; C. K. Scott, M. A. Foss, and M. L. Dennis, "Pathways in the Replace–Treatment–Recovery Cycle Over 3 Years," *Journal of Substance Abuse Treatment* 28 (2005): S63–S72; Philippe Bourgois and Jeffery Schonberg, *Righteous Dopefiend* (Berkeley: University of California Press, 2009).

31 Jeremy A. Greene, "Therapeutic Infidelities: 'Noncompliance' Enters the Medical Literature, 1955–1975," *Social History of Medicine* 17, no. 3 (2004): 327–43.

32 Charles Rosenberg, "Banishing Risk: Continuity and Change in the Moral Management of Disease," in *Morality and Health: Interdisciplinary Perspectives*, ed. A. Brandt and P. Rozin (New York: Routledge, 1997), 35–52.

33 Joan F. Epstein and Joseph C. Gfroerer, "Heroin abuse in the United States," Office of Applied Studies Substance Abuse and Mental Health Services Administration (1997). www.health.org.80/govpubs/Rpo919/index.htm (accessed 15 June 2007).

34 Drug Abuse Warning Network (DAWN), "Year Emergency Room Data from the Drug Abuse Warning Network," Substance Abuse and Mental Health Services Administration (SAMHSA), Office of Applied Studies, DAWN Series D-18 (2001), DHHS Publication No. (SMA) 01-3532.

35 L. A. Marsch, W. K. Bickel, G. J. Badger, and E. A. Jacobs, "Buprenorphine Treatment for Opioid Dependence: The Relative Efficacy of Daily, Twice and Thrice Weekly Dosing," *Drug and Alcohol Dependence* 77 (2005): 195–204.

36 D. H. Gandhi et al., "Short-Term Outcomes After Brief Ambulatory Opioid Detoxification with Buprenorphine in Young Heroin Users," *Addiction* 98 (2003): 453–62.

37 G. R. Zanni, "Review: Patient Diaries, Charting the Course," *Consultant Pharmacist* 22 (2007): 472–76, 479–82. Here the assumption is that clinical diaries provide a way for patients to assess their own health status without clinician bias or interpretation. The "chart" that Cedric and Megan kept was not, however, to

map symptoms or experiences unaccounted for in the chart at the clinic. Its significance exists outside of the document itself.

5 / Patienthood

1   François Dagognet, *La raison et les remèdes* (Paris: Presses Universitaires de France, 1964).

2   Byron Good, *Medicine, Rationality and Experience: An Anthropological Perspective* (Cambridge: Cambridge University Press, 1994).

3   G. Danzer, M. Rose, M. Walter, and B. F. Klapp, "On the Theory of Individual Health," *Journal of Medical Ethics* 28 (2002): 17–19; Lennart Nordenfelt, "On the Relevance and Importance of the Notion of Disease," *Theoretical Medicine* 14 (1993): 15–26; Christopher Boorse, "On the Distinction between Disease and Illness," *Philosophy and Public Affairs* 5, no. 1 (1975): 49–68; Christopher Boorse, "Health as a Theoretical Concept," *Philosophy of Science* 44, no. 4 (1977): 542–73; Élodie Giroux, *Après Canguilhem: Définir la santé et la maladie* (Paris: Presses Universitaires de France, 2010).

4   Mark Letteri, "The Theme of Health in Nietzsche's Thought," *Man and World* 23 (1990): 405–17.

5   Scott H. Podolsky and Alfred I. Tauber, "Nietzsche's Conception of Health: The Idealization of Struggle," in *Nietzsche, Epistemology, and Philosophy of Science: Nietzsche and the Sciences II*, ed. B. Babich (London: Kluwer, 1999).

6   Letteri, "Theme of Health," 410; Friedrich Nietzsche, *The Will to Power*, trans. Walter Kaufmann (New York: Vintage Books, 1968), 346.

7   Georges Canguilhem, "Health: Popular Concept and Philosophical Question," in *Writings on Medicine*, trans. Stefanos Geroulanos and Todd Meyers (New York: Fordham University Press, 2012), 43–52.

8   Robert Desjarlais offers a detailed analysis of the daily routine of the homeless shelter, and how these routines came to shape the subjectivity of the residents of the center, in *Shelter Blues: Sanity and Selfhood among the Homeless* (Philadelphia: University of Pennsylvania Press, 1997).

9   Philippe Bourgois and Jeff Schonberg, *Righteous Dopefiend* (Berkeley: University of California Press, 2009); Guillaume Le Blanc, *L'invisibilité sociale* (Paris: Presses Universitaires de France, 2009).

10 The issue here is a departure from what Allan Young describes as the advent of specific modes of diagnostics related to Post-Traumatic Stress Disorder (PTSD) in *The Harmony of Illusions: Inventing Post-Traumatic Stress Disorder* (Princeton, NJ: Princeton University Press, 1997).

11 See Canguilhem's long discussion of "the sick man" in *The Normal and the Pathological*, trans. C. Fawcett (New York: Zone Books, 1989), particularly the chapter entitled "Disease, Cure, Health," 181–201; see also Guillaume Le Blanc's discussion of Canguilhem's work in *Les maladies de l'homme normal* (Paris: J. Vrin, 2007).

12 Michel Foucault, *The Birth of the Clinic*, trans. A. M. Sheridan (New York: Vintage, 1973), 149.

13 Arthur Frank, *At the Will of the Body: Reflections on Illness* (Boston, MA: Houghton Mifflin Company, 1991), 58.

14 Canguilhem, *Writings on Medicine*, 34–35; see also Michel Foucault, "The Birth of Social Medicine," in *The Essential Works of Foucault, 1954–1984, Vol. III, Power*, trans. R. Hurley (New York: The New Press, 2000), 154–56.

15 Canguilhem, *The Normal and the Pathological*.

16 Virginia Woolf, *On Being Ill* (Ashfield, MA: Paris Press, 2002), 7.

17 The most detailed (and difficult) account is Jean-Luc Nancy's *L'Intrus* (Paris: Galilée, 2000); also see the new translation by Richard A. Rand of Nancy's essay in *Corpus* (New York: Fordham University Press, 2008).

18 Roy Porter, "The Patient's View: Doing Medical History from Below," *Theory and Society* 4 (1985): 175–98.

19 Shigehisa Kuriyama, *The Expressiveness of the Body and the Divergence of Greek and Chinese Medicine* (New York: Zone Books, 2002), 9.

20 Canguilhem, *The Normal and the Pathological*, 115.

21 Veena Das, "Sufferings, Theodicies, Disciplinary Practices, Appropriations," *International Social Science Journal/UNESCO* 49, no. 154 (1997): 563–72.

22 Luc Boltanski, *La découverte de la maladie: La diffusion du savior medical* (Paris: Centre de Sociologie Européenne, 1968).

23 Maurice Merleau-Ponty, *Consciousness and the Acquisition of Language*, trans. Hugh L. Silverman (Evanston, IL: Northwestern University Press, 1973), 10.

24 Gilbert Simondon. *L'individu et sa genèse physico-biologique: L'individuation à la lumière des notions de forme et d'information* (Paris: Presses Universitaires de France, 1964).

6 / Disappearances

1 Arthur Kleinman, *Writings at the Margin: Discourse between Anthropology and Medicine* (Berkeley: University of California Press, 1995).

2 Anand Pandian, "Interior Horizons: An Ethical Space of Selfhood in South India," *The Journal of the Royal Anthropological Institute* 16 (2010): 64–83.

3 Robert Desjarlais, *Shelter Blues: Sanity and Selfhood among the Homeless* (Philadelphia, PA: University of Pennsylvania Press, 1997), 248.

4 Michel Foucault, *The History of Sexuality, Vol. 3, The Care of the Self*, trans. Robert Hurley (New York: Pantheon, 1986).

5 Guillaume Le Blanc, *Les maladies de l'homme normal* (Paris: J. Vrin, 2007).

6 Gilles Deleuze, *Pure Immanence: Essay on A Life*, trans. Anne Boyman (New York: Zone Books, 2001).

7 See my introduction, "Life, as such" (with Paola Marrati), to Georges Canguilhem's *Knowledge of Life*, trans. Stefanos Geroulanos and Daniela Ginsberg (New

York: Fordham University Press, 2008), vii-xii.

8   François Dagognet, *La raison et les remèdes* (Paris: Presses Universitaires de France, 1964).

9   Canguilhem, *Knowledge of Life*.

10 Michel Foucault, "La vie: L'expérience et la science," *Revue de métaphysique et de morale* 90 (1985): 3–14.

11 Foucault, *The History of Sexuality, Vol. 3, The Care of the Self*.

12 Georges Canguilhem, "Health: Popular Concept and Philosophical Question," in *Writings on Medicine*, trans. Stefanos Geroulanos and Todd Meyers (New York: Fordham University Press, 2012), 43-52.

13 See, for instance, Sandra Laugier's discussion of Cavell and Austin, "Rethinking the Ordinary: Austin *after* Cavell," in *Contending with Stanley Cavell*, ed. Russell B. Goodman (New York: Oxford University Press, 2005), 82–99; and *Wittgenstein: Les sens de l'usage* (Paris: J. Vrin, 2009).

14 Pamela Reynolds's discussion of political conflict in South Africa rupturing the family unit and blocking relationships, only to remake and reform them, has aided my thoughts tremendously. Pamela Reynolds, "The Ground of All Making: State Violence, the Family, and Political Activists," in *Violence and Subjectivity*, ed. V. Das et al. (Berkeley: University of California Press, 1997), 141–207.

15 See Angela Garcia's excellent and eloquent work on intimacy and the reshaping of an ethics of care in families contending with heroin addiction, in *The Pastoral Clinic: Addiction and Dispossession along the Rio Grande* (Berkeley: University of California Press, 2010).

16 In Gilles Deleuze's discussion of Francois Bacon's paintings, the break with representation that Bacon makes disrupts the single thread of narration in order to "make shadows as present as the Figure," Gilles Deleuze, *Francis Bacon: Logic of Sensation*, trans. Daniel W. Smith (Minneapolis: University of Minnesota Press, 2006), 8.

Conclusion

1   Georges Canguilhem, *Writings on Medicine*, trans. Stefanos Geroulanos and Todd Meyers (New York: Fordham University Press, 2012), 66.

2   Samuel Beckett, *Proust* (New York: Grove Press, 1965), 19.

3   The core argument in Elaine Scarry's *The Body in Pain* (1985) is that pain defies language while unmaking worlds. However, there is something subtler here, particularly in Jeff's case. It is something that Veena Das, in an essay entitled "Language and Body: Transactions in the Constructions of Pain" from her *Life and Words: Violence and the Descent into the Ordinary* (Berkeley: University of California Press, 2007), describes beautifully and forcefully as the lack of a standing language of pain. The language offered through another's pain, something

nearly untroubled in the social sciences, attends to the transaction between language and body. There is no standing language of pain because, as Canguilhem asserts regarding the experience of illness by the "sick man," there is no access to "ordinary concepts." What Das suggests, however, does not fall in to the trap Susan Sontag lays for herself in her *Regarding the Pain of Others* (New York: Farrar, Straus and Giroux, 2003). The "modern" tendency to distance horror through the image is not an acknowledgment of the incapacity of one's language to act as a substitute for another's pain, but, as Sontag—seeming to hold a special ire for Georges Bataille—mistakenly identifies as an indiscriminate, collective appetite for showing bodies in pain in order to find transcendence, religious or otherwise.

4 Beckett, *Proust*, 13.
5 On the subject of clinical trials, see again Harry Marks, *The Progress of Experiment: Science and Therapeutic Reform in the United States, 1900–1990* (New York: Cambridge University Press, 1997).

Bibliography

Alvania, Rebecca. "Drug Disabuse: Bupe Treats Heroin Addiction Easily and Safely but Remains Hard to Come By." *The City Paper*, December 19, 2007.

Amato, L., S. Minozze, M. Davoli, S. Vecchi, M. M. Ferri, and S. Mayet. "Psychosocial and Pharmacological Treatments versus Pharmacological Treatments for Opioid Detoxification." *Cochrane Database Systematic Reviews* 3 (2008): CD005031.

Bachelard, Gaston. *The Poetics of Space*. Translated by M. Jolas. New York: Beacon Press, 1994.

Bailey, Katharine P. "Pharmacological Treatments for Substance Use Disorders." *Journal of Psychosocial Nursing* 42, no. 8 (2004): 14–20.

Baltimore City Council President. "City Council President Stephanie Rawlings-Blake Calls for Public Hearing on Heroin Treatment: President to Request Expansion on City's Buprenorphine Availability." Press release, March 26, 2007.

Bayer, Ronald, and David Wilkinson. "Directly Observed Therapy for Tuberculosis: History of an Idea." *Lancet* 345, no. 8964 (1995): 1545.

Becker, S. J., and J. F. Curry. "Outpatient Interventions for Adolescent Substance Abuse: A Quality of Evidence Review." *Journal of Consulting and Clinical Psychology* 76, no. 4 (2008): 531–43.

Beckett, Samuel. *Proust*. New York: Grove Press, 1965. First publication in French: London: Chatto & Windus, 1931.

Bickel, Warren K., Maxine L. Stitzer, George E. Bigelow, Ira A. Liebson, Donald R. Jasinski, and Rolley E. Johnson. "A Clinical Trial of Buprenorphine: Comparison with Methadone in the Detoxification of Heroin Addicts." *Clinical Pharmacology & Therapeutics* 43, no. 1 (1988): 72–78.

Biehl, João. *Will to Live: AIDS Therapies and the Politics of Survival*. Princeton, NJ: Princeton University Press, 2007.

Biehl, João, and Amy Moran-Thomas. "Symptom: Subjectivities, Social Ills, Technologies." *Annual Review of Anthropology* 38 (2009): 267–88.

Boltanski, Luc. *La découverte de la maladie: La diffusion du savoir médical*. Paris: Centre de Sociologie Européenne, 1968.

Boorse, Christopher. "On the Distinction between Disease and Illness." *Philosophy and Public Affairs* 5, no. 1 (1975): 49–68.

———. "Health as a Theoretical Concept." *Philosophy of Science* 44, no. 4 (1977): 542–73.

Bourgois, Philippe. "Intimate Apartheid: Ethnic Dimensions of Habitus Among Homeless Heroin Injectors." *Ethnography* 8, no. 1 (2007): 7–31.

Bourgois, Philippe, and Jeffery Schonberg. *Righteous Dopefiend*. Berkeley: University of California Press, 2009.

Brandt, Allan. "Behavior, Disease, and Health in the Twentieth-Century United States: The Moral Valence of Individual Risk." In *Morality and Health: Interdisciplinary Perspectives*, edited by A. Brandt and P. Rozin, 53–78. New York: Routledge, 1997.

Braunstein, Jean-François, ed. *Canguilhem, histoire des sciences et politique du vivant*. Paris: Presses Universitaires de France, 2007.

Brown, Truesdell S. *Timaeus of Tauromenium*. Berkeley: University of California Press, 1958.

Campbell, Nancy. *Discovering Addiction: The Science and Politics of Substance Abuse Research*. Ann Arbor: University of Michigan Press, 2007.

Campbell, Nancy, and Anne M. Lovell. "The History of the Development of Buprenorphine as an Addiction Therapeutic." *Annals of the New York Academy of Sciences* 1248 (2012): 124–39.

Campbell, Nancy, and Susan Shaw. "Incitements to Discourse: Illicit Drugs, Harm Reduction, and the Production of Ethnographic Subjects." *Cultural Anthropology* 23, no. 4 (2009): 688–717.

Canguilhem, Georges. *Études d'histoire et de philosophie des sciences*. Paris: J. Vrin, 1968.

———. *The Normal and the Pathological*. Translated by C. Fawcett. New York: Zone Books, 1989.

———. *Knowledge of Life*. Edited by Paola Marrati and Todd Meyers. Translated by Stefanos Geroulanos and Daniela Ginsburg. New York: Fordham University Press, 2008.

———. *Writings on Medicine*. Translated by Stefanos Geroulanos and Todd Meyers. New York: Fordham University Press, 2012.

Carr, E. Summerson. *Scripting Addiction: The Politics of Therapeutic Talk and American Sobriety*. Princeton, NJ: Princeton University Press, 2010.

Castel, Robert. *La gestion des risques*. Paris: Les Editions du Minuit, 1981.

Cavell, Stanley. *Little Did I Know: Excerpts from Memory*. Palo Alto, CA: Stanford University Press, 2010.

Center for a Healthy Maryland. "Report: Improving Patient Access to Buprenorphine Treatment through Physician Offices in Maryland." June 2007, http://www.healthymaryland.org/substance-use-buprenorphine.php (accessed 11 August 2007).

Chatterji, Roma. "An Ethnography of Dementia." *Culture, Medicine, & Psychiatry* 22, no. 3 (1988): 355–82.

Clemmey, P., L. Payne, H. Adger, and M. Fishman. *Manual for a Short-term Residential Treatment Program for Adolescent Substance Use Disorders* (title amended). Bloomington, IL: Chestnut Health Systems, 2003.

Clemmey, P., L. Payne, and M. Fishman. "Clinical Characteristics and Treatment Outcomes of Adolescent Heroin Users." *Journal of Psychoactive Drugs* 36 (2004): 85–94.

Courtwright, David. *Dark Paradise: A History of Opiate Addiction in America.* Cambridge, MA: Harvard University Press, 2001.

Cowan, Alan, and John W. Lewis, eds. *Buprenorphine: Combating Drug Abuse with a Unique Opioid.* New York: Wiley-Liss Publications, 1995.

Dagognet, François. *La raison et les remèdes.* Paris: Presses Universitaires de France, 1964.

Dahl, R. E., and L. P. Spear, eds. *Adolescent Brain Development: Vulnerabilities and Opportunities. Annals of the New York Academy of Sciences* 1021 (2004): 1–469.

Daly, Jeanne. *Evidence-Based Medicine and the Search for a Science of Clinical Care.* Berkeley: University of California Press, 2005.

Danzer, G., M. Rose, M. Walter, and B. F. Klapp. "On the theory of individual health." *Journal of Medical Ethics* 28 (2002): 17–19.

Das, Veena. "Sufferings, Theodicies, Disciplinary Practices, Appropriations." *International Social Science Journal/UNESCO* 49, no. 154 (1997): 563–72.

———. *Life and Words: Violence and the Descent into the Ordinary.* Berkeley: University of California Press, 2007.

Das, V., A. Kleinman, M. Ramphele, and P. Reynolds, ed. *Violence and Subjectivity.* Berkeley: University of California Press, 1997.

Day, E., J. Ison, and J. Strang. "Inpatient versus Other Settings for Detoxification for Opioid Dependence." *Cochrane Database of Systematic Reviews* 2 (2005): CD004580.

Deleuze, Gilles. *Pure Immanence: Essays on A Life.* Translated by Anne Boyman. New York: Zone Books, 2001.

———. *Francis Bacon: Logic of Sensation.* Translated by Daniel W. Smith. Minneapolis: University of Minnesota Press, 2006.

Derrida, Jacques. *Archive Fever.* Translated by Eric Prenowitz. Chicago: University of Chicago Press, 1995.

Desjarlais, Robert. *Shelter Blues: Sanity and Selfhood among the Homeless.* Philadelphia: University of Pennsylvania Press, 1997.

Ditkoff, Anna. "Bloodletting: Can Anything Be Done to Bring Baltimore's Homicide Rate Down?" *The City Paper*, January 23, 2008.

Donaher, P. A., and C. Welsh. "Managing Opioid Addiction with Buprenorphine: Review." *American Family Physician* 73, no. 9 (2006): 1573–78.

Donovan, Doug, and Fred Schulte. "Not a Cure-all: Despite Praise, 'Bupe' Alone Isn't Enough to Break Addicts of Destructive Routines." *The Baltimore Sun*, December 18, 2007.

———. "Bupe Seizures Rise as Treatment Use Grows." *The Baltimore Sun*, April 18, 2008.

Doron, Olivier, Céline Lefève, and Alain-Charles Masquelet, eds. *Soin et subjectivité.* Paris: Presses Universitaires de France, 2010.

Drug Abuse Warning Network (DAWN). "Year Emergency Room Data from the Drug Abuse Warning Network." Substance Abuse and Mental Health Services Administration (SAMHSA), Office of Applied Studies, DAWN Series D-18 (2001), DHHS Publication No. (SMA) 01-3532.

Epstein, Joan F., and Joseph C. Gfroerer. "Heroin Abuse in the United States." Office of Applied Studies Substance Abuse and Mental Health Services Administration (1997). www.health.org.80/govpubs/Rp0919/index.htm (accessed 15 June 2007).

Epstein, Steven. *Inclusion: The Politics of Difference in Medical Research.* Chicago: University of Chicago Press, 2007.

Esposito, Roberto. *Bíos: Biopolitics and Philosophy.* Translated by Timothy Campbell. Minneapolis: University of Minnesota Press, 2008.

Farmer, Paul, et al. "Letter to the Editor: Directly Observed Therapy for HIV Anti-Retroviral Therapy in an Urban U.S. Setting." *Journal of Acquired Immune Deficiencies Syndrome* 36, no. 91 (2004): 642–44.

Federal Register. "Buprenorphine Prescribing Practices Survey." Vol. 67, no. 233 (2002): 72219.

———. "Meeting on Buprenorphine Treatment." Vol. 67, no. 175 (2002): 57445.

Feroni, Isabelle, and Anne M. Lovell. "Les dispositifs de regulation publique d'un medicament sensible: Le cas du Subutex®, traitement de substitution aux opiaces." *Revue française des affaires sociales. Cahier de jurisprudence. Emploi-travail* 61, no. 3 (2007): 153–65.

Fiellin, David A. "The First Three Years of Buprenorphine in the United States: Experience to Date and Future Directions." *Journal of Addiction Medicine* 1, no. 2 (2007): 62–67.

———. "Treatment of Adolescent Opioid Dependence: No Quick Fix." *Journal of the American Medical Association* 300, no. 17 (2008): 2057–59.

Fiellin, David A., and Patrick G. O'Connor. "New Federal Initiatives to Enhance the Medical Treatment of Opioid Dependence." *Annals of Internal Medicine* 137, no. 8 (2002): 688–92.

———. "Office-Based Treatment of Opioid-Dependent Patients." *New England Journal of Medicine* 347 (2002): 817–23.

Fiellin, David A., Robert A. Rosenheck, and Thomas R. Kosten. "Office-Based Treatment for Opioid Dependence: Reaching New Patient Populations." *American Journal of Psychiatry* 158 (2001): 1200–204.

Fishman, M., A. Bruner, and H. Adger. "Substance Abuse among Children and Adolescents." *Pediatric Review* 18 (1997): 394–403.

Fleck, Ludwik. *Genèse et développement d'un fait scientifique* (Genesis and development of a scientific fact). Translated by Nathalie Jas. Paris: Flammarion, 2008.

Food and Drug Administration. "Subutex and Suboxone Approved to Treat Opiate Dependence." Press release, October 2, 2002.

———. "Drug Shortage: Drug to be Discontinued Letter from Roxane (ORLAAM

[Levomethadyl hydrochloride acetate] Solution)." Press release, August 23, 2003.

Foucault, Michel. *The Birth of the Clinic.* Translated by A. Sheridan. New York: Vintage, 1973.

———. *Discipline and Punish: The Birth of the Prison.* Translated by A. Sheridan. New York: Vintage, 1977.

———. *Dits et Écrits: 1954–1975.* Paris: Gallimard, 1978.

———. "La vie: L'expérience et la science." *Revue de métaphysique et de morale* 90 (1985): 3–14.

———. *The History of Sexuality, Vol. 3, The Care of the Self.* Translated by Robert Hurley. New York: Pantheon, 1986.

———. "Technologies of the Self." In *Technologies of the Self,* edited by L. H. Martin, H. Gutman, and P. H. Hutton, 16–49. Amherst: University of Massachusetts Press, 1988.

———. "The Ethics of the Concern for Self as a Practice of Freedom." Translated by R. Hurley. In *The Essential Works of Foucault, 1954–1984, Vol. I, Ethics: Subjectivity and Truth,* edited by P. Rabinow, 281–302. New York: The New Press, 1997.

———. "The Birth of Social Medicine." In *The Essential Works of Foucault, 1954–1984, Vol. III, Power,* 154–56. Edited by P. Rabinow. Translated by R. Hurley. New York: The New Press, 2000.

Frank, Arthur. *At the Will of the Body: Reflections on Illness.* Boston, MA: Houghton Mifflin Company, 1991.

———. "Stories of Illness as Care of the Self: A Foucauldian Dialogue." *Health* 2 (1998): 329.

Fudala, Paul J., Jerome H. Jaffe, Elizabeth M. Dax, and Rolley E. Johnson. "Use of Buprenorphine in the Treatment of Opioid Addiction: II. Physiologic and Behavioral Effects of Daily and Alternate-day Administration and Abrupt Withdrawal." *Clinical Pharmacology & Therapeutics* 47, no. 4 (1990): 525–34.

Gaertner, J., R. Voltz, and C. Ostgathe. "Methadone: A Closer Look at the Controversy." *Journal of Pain Symptom Management* 36, no. 2 (2008): e4–e7.

Gandhi, D. H., J. H. Jaffe, S. McNary, G. Kavanagh, M. Hayes, and M. Currens. "Short-Term Outcomes After Brief Ambulatory Opioid Detoxification with Buprenorphine in Young Heroin Users." *Addiction* 98 (2003): 453–62.

Gandhi, D. H., G. J. Kavanagh, and J. H. Jaffe. "Young Heroin Users in Baltimore: A Qualitative Study." *American Journal of Drug and Alcohol Abuse* 32 (2006): 177–88.

Garcia, Angela. *The Pastoral Clinic: Addiction and Dispossession along the Rio Grande.* Berkeley: University of California Press, 2010.

Gardner, Robert. *Making Forest of Bliss: Intention, Circumstance, and Chance in Nonfiction Film.* Cambridge, MA: Harvard Film Archive, 2001.

Garrau, Marie, and Alice Le Goff. *Care, justice, dépendance: Introduction aux théories du care.* Paris: Presses Universitaires de France, 2010.

Geertz, Clifford. *The Interpretation of Cultures.* New York: Basic Books, 1973.

Gilligan, Carol. *In a Different Voice: Psychological Theory and Women's Development.*

Cambridge, MA: Harvard University Press, 1983.

Giroux, Élodie. *Après Canguilhem: Définir la santé et la maladie.* Paris: Presses Universitaires de France, 2010.

Goldstein, Kurt. *The Organism.* New York: Zone Books, 1995.

Goffman, Erving. *Forms of Talk.* Philadelphia: University of Pennsylvania Press, 1981.

Good, Byron. *Medicine, Rationality and Experience: An Anthropological Perspective.* Cambridge, MA: Cambridge University Press, 1994.

Gowing, L., and A. White. "Buprenorphine for the Management of Opioid Dependence: Review." *Cochrane Database of Systematic Reviews* 2, no. 3 (2006): CD002025.

Greene, Jeremy A. "Therapeutic Infidelities: Noncompliance Enters the Medical Literature: 1955–1975." *Social History of Medicine* 17, no. 3 (2004): 327–43.

———. *Prescribing by Numbers: Drugs and the Definition of Disease.* Baltimore, MD: Johns Hopkins University Press, 2007.

Jaffe, Jerome H., and Charles O'Keeffe. "From Morphine Clinics to Buprenorphine: Regulating Opioid Agonist Treatment of Addiction in the United States." *Drug and Alcohol Dependence* 70 (2003): S3–S11.

Jasinski, D. R., J. S. Pevnick, and J. D. Griffith. "Human Pharmacology and Abuse Potential of the Analgesic Buprenorphine: A Potential Agent for Treating Narcotic Addiction." *Archives of General Psychiatry* 35, no. 4 (1978): 501–16.

Jenkins, Janis H., ed. *Pharmaceutical Self: The Global Shaping of Experience in an Age of Psychopharmacology.* Santa Fe, NM: School for Advanced Research Press, 2012.

Jernigan, T. L., et al. "Maturation of Human Cerebrum Observed in vivo During Adolescence." *Brain* 114 (1991): 2037–49.

Johnson, Rolley E. "Letter from Reckitt Benckiser VP for Scientific and Regulatory Affairs." *The Baltimore Sun*, December 17, 2007.

Johnson, Rolley E., Edward J. Cone, Jack E. Henningfield, and Paul J. Fudala. "Use of Buprenorphine in the Treatment of Opiate Addiction. I. Physiologic and Behavioral Effects During a Rapid Dose Induction." *Clinical Pharmacology & Therapeutics* 46, no. 3 (1989): 335–43.

Johnson, Rolley E., Thomas Eissenberg, Maxine L. Stitzer, Eric C. Strain, Ira A. Liebson, and George E. Bigelow. "A Placebo Controlled Clinical Trial of Buprenorphine as a Treatment for Opioid Dependence." *Drug and Alcohol Dependence* 40 (1995): 17–25.

Johnson, Rolley E., Jerome H. Jaffe, and Paul J. Fudala. "A Controlled Trial of Buprenorphine Treatment for Opioid Dependence." *Journal of the American Medical Association* 267, no. 20 (1992): 2750–55.

Johnson, Rolley E., Eric C. Strain, and Leslie Amass. "Review: Buprenorphine, How to Use It Right." *Drug and Alcohol Dependence* 70 (2003): S59–S77.

Johnston, L. D., P. M. O'Malley, J. G. Bachman, and J. E. Schulenberg. *Monitoring the Future: National Survey Results on Drug Use, 1975–2007. Vol. I, Secondary School Students* (NIH Publication No. 08–6418A). Bethesda, MD: National Institute on Drug Abuse, 2007.

Jones, Jill. *Hep-Cats, Narcs, and Pipe Dreams: A History of America's Romance with Illegal Drugs*. Baltimore, MD: Johns Hopkins University Press, 1999.

Jorland, G., A. Opinel, and G. Weisz, eds. *Body Counts: Medical Quantification in Historical and Sociological Perspectives*. Montreal: McGill-Queen's University Press, 2005.

Joseph, H., S. Stancliff, and J. Langrod. "Methadone Maintenance Treatment (MMT): A Review of Historical and Clinical Issues." *Mt. Sinai Journal of Medicine* 67, no. 5-6 (2000): 347–64.

Kleber, Herbert D. "Naltrexone." *Journal of Substance Abuse Treatment* 2 (1985): 117–22.

Kleber, Herbert D. "Methadone Maintenance Four Decades Later: Thousands of Lives Saved but Still Controversial." *Journal of the American Medical Association* 300, no. 19 (2008): 2303–05.

Kleinman, Arthur. *The Illness Narratives: Suffering, Healing, and the Human Condition*. New York: Basic Books, 1987.

———. *Writings at the Margin: Discourse between Anthropology and Medicine*. Berkeley: University of California Press, 1995.

Knudsen, H. K., L. J. Ducharme, and P. M. Roman. "Early Adoption of Buprenorphine in Substance Abuse Treatment Centers: Data from the Private and Public Sectors." *Journal of Substance Abuse and Treatment* 30, no. 4 (2006): 363–73.

Koch, Alison L., Cynthia L. Arfken, and Charles R. Schuster. "Characteristics of U.S. Substance Abuse Treatment Facilities Adopting Buprenorphine in Its Initial Stage of Availability." *Drug and Alcohol Dependence* 83, no. 3 (2006): 274–78.

Kosten, Thomas R., and Tony P. George. "The Neurobiology of Opioid Dependence: Implications for Treatment." *Science & Practice Perspectives* 1, no. 1 (2002): 13–20.

Kosten, Thomas R., Charles Morgan, and Herbert O. Kleber. "Phase II Clinical Trials of Buprenorphine: Detoxification and Induction onto Naltrexone." *NIDA Monograph* 121 (1992): 101–19.

Kreek, Mary Jeanne. "Methadone-Related Opioid Agonist Pharmacotherapy for Heroin Addiction: History, Recent Molecular and Neuro-chemical Research and Future in Mainstream Medicine." *Annals of the New York Academy of Sciences* 909 (2000): 186–216.

Kreek, Mary Jeanne, and Frank J. Vocci. "History and Current Status of Opioid Maintenance Treatments: Blending Conference Session." *Journal of Substance Abuse Treatment* 23 (2002): 93–105.

Kuriyama, Shigehisa. *The Expressiveness of the Body in Greek and Chinese Medicine*. New York: Zone Books, 2000.

Lakoff, Andrew. *Pharmaceutical Reason: Knowledge and Value in Global Psychiatry*. New York: Cambridge University Press, 2006.

Laugier, Sandra. "Rethinking the Ordinary: Austin *after* Cavell." In *Contending with Stanley Cavell*, edited by Russell B. Goodman, 82–99. New York: Oxford University Press, 2005.

———. "Wittgenstein and Cavell: Anthropology, Skepticism, and Politics." In *The Claim to Community: Essays on Stanley Cavell and Political Philosophy*, edited by

Andrew Norris, 19–37. Palo Alto, CA: Stanford University Press, 2006.

———. *Wittgenstein: Les sens de l'usage*. Paris: J. Vrin, 2009.

Le Blanc, Guillaume. *Les maladies de l'homme normal*. Paris: J. Vrin, 2007.

———. *L'invisibilité sociale*. Paris: Presses Universitaires de France, 2009.

Leonard, Lori, and Jonathan Ellen. "'The Story of My Life': AIDS and Autobiographical Occasions." *Qualitative Sociology* 31, no. 1 (2008): 37–56.

Letteri, Mark. "The Theme of Health in Nietzsche's Thought." *Man and World* 23 (1990): 405–17.

Levin, Carl. Congressional Record—Senate, and Commentaries, S1091–S1093, January 28, 1999.

———. "FDA Approval of Buprenorphine." Press Release, October 9, 2002.

———. "FDA Approval of Medication to Combat Heroin Addiction Culminates Long-Fought Battle, Says Levin." Press release, October 9, 2002.

Lewis, Gilbert. *A Failure of Treatment*. New York: Oxford University Press, 2000.

Lewis, J. W., and D. Walter. "Buprenorphine: Background to Its Development as a Treatment for Opiate Dependence." *NIDA Monograph* 21 (1992): 5–11.

Ling, Walter, and Donald R. Wesson. "Clinical Efficacy of Buprenorphine: Comparisons to Methadone and Placebo." *Drug and Alcohol Dependence* 70 (2003): S49–S57.

Ling, Walter, Leslie Amass, Steve Shoptaw, Jeffrey J. Annon, et al. "A Multi-Center Randomized Trial of Buprenorphine-Naloxone versus Clonidine for Opioid Detoxification: Findings from the National Institute on Drug Abuse Clinical Trials Network." *Addiction* 100 (2005): 1090–1100.

Lipman, A. G. "Methadone: Effective Analgesia, Confusion, and Risk." *Journal of Pain & Palliative Care Pharmacotherapy* 19 (2005): 3–5.

Lopez, B., S. J. Schwartz, G. Prado, A. E. Campo, and H. Pantin. "Adolescent Neurological Development and Its Implications for Adolescent Substance Abuse Prevention." *Journal of Primary Prevention* 29, no. 1 (2008): 5–35.

Lovell, Anne M. "Ordonner les risques: L'individu et le pharmaco-sociatif face à la réduction des dommages dans l'injection de drogues." In *Critique de la santé publique: Une approche anthropologique*, edited by Jean-Pierre Dozon and Didier Fassin, 309–42. Paris: Balland, 2001.

———. "Addiction Markets: The Case of High-dose Buprenorphine in France." In *Global Pharmaceuticals*, edited by Adriana Petryna, Andrew Lakoff, and Arthur Kleinman, 136–70. Durham, NC: Duke University Press, 2006.

Marks, Harry. *The Progress of Experiment: Science and Therapeutic Reform in the United States, 1900–1990*. New York: Cambridge University Press, 1997.

Marsch, L. A., W. K. Bickel, G. J. Badger, and E. A. Jacobs. "Buprenorphine Treatment for Opioid Dependence: The Relative Efficacy of Daily, Twice and Thrice Weekly Dosing." *Drug and Alcohol Dependence* 77 (2005): 195–204.

Marsch, L. A., W. K. Bickel, G. J. Badger, M. E. Stothart, et al. "Comparison of Pharmacological Treatments for Opioid-Dependent Adolescents." *Archives of General Psychiatry* 62, no. 10 (2005): 1157–64.

Matthews, R. J. *Quantification and the Quest for Medical Certainty*. Princeton, NJ: Princeton University Press, 1995.

McClellan, Mark B. "Two Drugs for Opioid Dependence." *Journal of the American Medical Association* 288, no. 21 (2002): 2678.

McCormick, Cynthia G., Jack E. Henningfield, J. David Haddox, Sajan Varughese, Anders Lindholm, Susan Rosen, Janne Wissel, Deborah Waxman, Lawrence P. Carter, Vickie Seeger, and Rolley E. Johnson. "Case Histories in Pharmaceutical Risk Management." *Drug and Alcohol Dependence* 105S (2009): S42-S55.

McLean, Athena, and Annette Leibing, eds. *Shadow Side: Exploring the Blurred Borders between Ethnography and Life*. Oxford, UK: Blackwell Publishing, 2007.

McMurphy, Suzanne, et al. "Clinic-Based Treatment for Opioid Dependence: A Qualitative Inquiry." *American Journal of Health Behavior* 30, no. 6 (2006): 544–54.

Meier, B. R., and A. A. Patkar. "Buprenorphine Treatment: Factors and First-hand Experiences for Providers to Consider." *Journal of Addictive Diseases* 26, no. 1 (2007): 3–14.

Merleau-Ponty, Maurice. *The Structure of Behavior*. Translated by Alden L. Fisher. New York: Beacon Press, 1963.

———. *The Visible and the Invisible*. Translated by Alphonso Lingis. Evanston, IL: Northwestern University Press, 1968.

———. *Consciousness and the Acquisition of Language*. Translated by Hugh L. Silverman. Evanston, IL: Northwestern University Press, 1973.

Meyers, Todd. "A Turn towards Dying: Presence, Signature, and the Social Course of Chronic Illness in Urban America." *Medical Anthropology* 26 (2007): 205–27.

Meyers, Todd, Lori Leonard, and Jonathan M. Ellen. "The Clinic and Elsewhere: Illness, Sexuality and Social Experience among Young African-American Men in Baltimore, Maryland." *Culture, Medicine, & Psychiatry* 28, no. 1 (2004): 67–86.

Mol, Annemarie. *The Logic of Care: Health and the Problem of Patient Choice*. London: Routledge, 2008.

Molinier, Pascale, Sandra Laugier, and Patricia Paperman, eds. *Qu'est-ce que le care?: Souci des autres, sensibilité, responsabilité*. Paris: Payot, 2009.

Morris, Diana. "Addiction Poses Greater Dangers." Letter to the editor, *The Baltimore Sun*, December 22, 2007.

Moshman, David. *Adolescent Rationality and Development: Cognition, Morality, Identity*. 3rd ed. New York: Psychology Press, 2011.

Nancy, Jean-Luc. *L'Intrus*. Paris: Galilée, 2000.

———. *Corpus*. Translated by Richard Rand. New York: Fordham University Press, 2008.

National Institutes of Health. "Hearing before the Health, Education, Labor, and Pensions Committee United States Senate: 'Oxycontin, Balancing Risks and Benefits.'" Statement of record, February 12, 2002.

———. "Buprenorphine Approval Expands Options for Addiction Treatment." *National Institute on Drug Abuse Research News* 17, no. 4 (2002).

Niedowski, Erika. "Success, Setbacks in France, French Approach to Drug Offers Lessons that U.S. Has Largely Overlooked." *The Baltimore Sun*, December 17, 2007.

Nietzsche, Friedrich. *The Gay Science*. Translated by Walter Kaufmann. New York: Vintage Books, 1974. (Originally published 1882.)

———. *The Will to Power*. Translated by Walter Kaufmann. New York: Vintage Books, 1968.

Nguyen, Vinh-Kim. *The Republic of Therapy: Triage and Sovereignty in West Africa's Time of AIDS*. Durham, NC: Duke University Press, 2010.

Nordenfelt, Lennart. "On the Relevance and Importance of the Notion of Disease." *Theoretical Medicine* 14 (1993): 15–26.

Nurock, Vanessa, ed. *Carol Gilligan et l'éthique du care*. Paris: Presses Universitaires de France, 2010.

O'Connor, Patrick G., et al. "Three Methods of Opioid Detoxification in a Primary Care Setting: A Randomized Trial." *Annals of Internal Medicine* 127, no. 7 (1997): 526–30.

———. "A Randomized Trial of Buprenorphine Maintenance for Heroin Dependence in a Primary Care Clinic for Substance Users versus a Methadone Clinic." *American Journal of Medicine* 105 (1998): 100–105.

O'Neil, John. "Vital Signs: A New Drug Means a New Venue." *New York Times*, October 15, 2002.

Pandian, Anand. "Interior Horizons: An Ethical Space of Selfhood in South India." *The Journal of the Royal Anthropological Institute* 16 (2010): 64–83.

Pandolfo, Stefania. *Impasse of the Angels: Scenes from a Moroccan Space of Memory*. Chicago: University of Chicago Press, 1997.

Pérez-Peña, Richard. "New Drug Promises Shift in Treatment for Heroin Addicts." *New York Times*, August 11, 2003.

Petryna, Adriana. "Ethical Variability: Drug Development and Globalizing Clinical Trials." *American Ethnologist* 32, no. 2 (2005): 183–97.

———. *When Experiments Travel: Clinical Trials and the Global Search for Human Subjects*. Princeton, NJ: Princeton University Press, 2009.

Petryna, Adriana, Andrew Lakoff, and Arthur Kleinman, eds. *Global Pharmaceuticals: Ethics, Markets, Practices*. Durham, NC: Duke University Press, 2006.

Pierron, Jean-Philippe. *Vulnérabilité: Pour une philosophie du soin*. Paris: Presses Universitaires de France, 2010.

Podolsky, Scott H., and Alfred I. Tauber. "Nietzsche's Conception of Health: The Idealization of Struggle." In *Nietzsche, Epistemology, and Philosophy of Science: Nietzsche and the Sciences II*, edited by B. Babich, 299–311. London: Kluwer, 1999.

Porter, Roy. "The Patient's View: Doing Medical History from Below." *Theory & Society* 4 (1985): 175–98.

Reckitt Benckiser Pharmaceuticals. "First New Addiction Treatment Products in 30 Years Approved for In-Office Treatment." Press release, October 9, 2002.

———. "Bush Signs Law: More Patients May Be Treated for Opioid Dependence/

Addiction with Buprenorphine." *Medical News Today*, January 2, 2007.

———. "Reckitt Benckiser Pharmaceuticals Inc. Receives FDA Approval for Sub-oxone® (Buprenorphine and Naloxone) Sublingual Film C-III." Press release, August 31, 2010.

Reynolds, Pamela. "The Ground of All Making: State Violence, the Family, and Political Activists." In *Violence and Subjectivity*, edited by V. Das, A. Kleinman, M. Ramphele and P. Reynolds, 141–207. Berkeley: University of California Press, 1997.

Rose, Nikolas. *The Politics of Life Itself: Biomedicine, Power, and Subjectivity in the Twenty-First Century*. Princeton, NJ: Princeton University Press, 2006.

Rosenberg, Charles. "Banishing Risk: Continuity and Change in the Moral Management of Disease." In *Morality and Health: Interdisciplinary Perspectives*, edited by A. Brandt and P. Rozin, 35–52. New York: Routledge, 1997.

Scarry, Elaine. *The Body in Pain: The Making and Unmaking of the World*. New York: Oxford University Press, 1985.

Schulte, Fred, and Doug Donovan. "The 'Bupe' Fix, Promoted by the U.S. as a Treatment for Opiate Addiction, Buprenorphine Has Become One More Item for Sale in the Illegal Drug Market." *The Baltimore Sun*, December 16, 2007.

———. "Drug Earning Millions Despite 'Orphan' Label: Status Granted before Law Increased Use of 'Bupe.'" *The Baltimore Sun*, December 18, 2007.

———. "Senators Urge Action to Reduce 'Bupe' Abuse, in MD, Lawmakers Vow Probe of State's Spending for Drug." *The Baltimore Sun*, December 20, 2007.

———. "Misuse of 'Bupe' Is Found to Be on the Rise, Report Shows: U.S. Could Exert Controls if Problem Deemed Serious." *The Baltimore Sun*, February 3, 2008.

———. "Strategies to Control Bupe Abuse Outlined." *The Baltimore Sun*, February 23, 2008.

Schuster, Charles R. "Conversation with Charles R. Schuster." *Addiction* 99, no. 6 (2004): 667–76.

Scott, C. K., M. A. Foss, and M. L. Dennis. "Pathways in the Replace–Treatment–Recovery Cycle Over 3 Years." *Journal of Substance Abuse Treatment* 28 (2005): S63–S72.

Serres, Michel. *The Five Senses: The Philosophy of Mingled Bodies*. New York: Continuum Press, 2009.

Sharfstein, Joshua, and Peter Luongo. "Addiction Poses Greater Dangers." Letter to the editor, *The Baltimore Sun*, December 22, 2007.

Simondon, Gilbert. *L'individu et sa genèse physic-biologique: L'individuation à la lumière des notions de forme et d'information*. Paris: Presses Universitaires de France, 1964.

Smith, Daniel W. "Deleuze on Bacon: Three Conceptual Trajectories in *The Logic of Sensation*." In *Francois Bacon: The Logic of Sensation*, by Gilles Deleuze, translated by Daniel W. Smith, vii-xxvii. Minneapolis: University of Minnesota Press, 2006.

Sontag, Susan. *Regarding the Pain of Others*. New York: Farrar, Straus & Giroux, 2003.

Spiller, Henry, et al. "Epidemiological Trends in Abuse and Misuse of Prescription Opioids." *Journal of Additive Diseases* 28, no. 2 (2009): 130–36.

Substance Abuse and Mental Health Service Administration. "Diversion and Abuse of Buprenorphine: A Brief Assessment of Emerging Indicators." December 2006. http://buprenorphine.samhsa.gov/Buprenorphine_FinalReport_12.6.06.pdf (accessed 2 July 2008).

———. "Buprenorphine: Patient Limits Increase," *SAMHSA News* January/February 2007.

Sullivan, L. E., and D. A. Fiellin. "Narrative Review: Buprenorphine for Opioid-Dependent Patients in Office Practice." *Annals of Internal Medicine* 148, no. 9 (2008): 662–70.

Taussig, Michael. *I Swear I Saw This: Drawings in Fieldwork Notebooks, Namely My Own.* Chicago: University of Chicago Press, 2011.

Tetrault, J. M., and D. A. Fiellin. "Current and Potential Pharmacological Treatment Options for Maintenance Therapy in Opioid-Dependent Individuals." *Drugs* 72, no. 2 (2012): 217–28.

Turner, Barbara J., et al. "Barriers and Facilitators to Primary Care or Human Immunodeficiency Virus Clinics Providing Methadone or Buprenorphine for the Management of Opioid Dependence." *Archives of Internal Medicine* 165 (2005): 1769–76.

United States Department of Justice, Drug Enforcement Administration, Office of Diversion Control. "Schedule of Controlled Substances: Proposed Rule: Rescheduling Buprenorphine from Schedule V to Schedule III." Press release, March 21, 2002.

United States House of Representatives. *Drug Addiction Treatment Act of 1999: Report Together with Additional Views (to accompany H.R. 2634; including cost estimate of the Congressional Budget Office).* Washington, D.C.: Government Printing Office, 1999.

Volkow, N. D. "What Do We Know About Drug Addiction?" *American Journal of Psychiatry* 162 (2005): 1401–02.

Wallace, John M., Jr., and Jerald G. Bachman. "Explaining Racial/Ethnic Differences in Adolescent Drug Use: The Impact of Background and Lifestyle." *Social Problems* 38, no. 3 (1991): 333–57.

Walsh, Sharon L., and Thomas Eissenberg. "The Clinical Pharmacology of Buprenorphine: Extrapolating from the Laboratory to the Clinic." *Drug and Alcohol Dependence* 70 (2003): S13–S27.

Welsh, Christopher. "Addiction Poses Greater Dangers." Letter to the editor, *The Baltimore Sun*, December 22, 2007.

Weisz, George. *Divide and Conquer: A Comparative History of Medical Specialization.* New York: Oxford University Press, 2006.

Wish, E. D., et al. "The Emerging Buprenorphine Epidemic in the United States." *Journal of Addictive Diseases* 31, no. 1 (2012): 3–7.

Woody, George E., Sabrina A. Poole, Geetha Subramaniam, et al. "Extended vs. Short-term Buprenorphine-Naloxone for Treatment of Opioid-Addicted Youth: A Randomized Trial." *Journal of the American Medical Association* 300, no. 17 (2008):

2003–11.

Woolf, Virginia. *On Being Ill*. New York: Paris Press, 2002. First edition: London: Hogarth Press, 1930.

Worms, Frédéric. *Le moment du soin*. Paris: Presses Universitaires de France, 2010.

Worms, Frédéric, Céline Lefève, Lazare Benaroyo, and Jean-Christophe Mino, eds. *La philosophie du soin*. Paris: Presses Universitaires de France, 2010.

Wren, Christopher S. "In Battle against Heroin, Scientists Enlist Heroin." *New York Times*, June 8, 1999.

Young, Allan. *The Harmony of Illusions: Inventing Post-Traumatic Stress Disorder*. Princeton, NJ: Princeton University Press, 1997.

Zanni, G. R. "Review: Patient Diaries, Charting the Course." *Consultant Pharmacist* 22 (2007): 472–76, 479–82.

INDEX